Anti-infective Guidelines for Community-acquired Infections

1997 - 2nd Edition - Revised

Ontario Anti-infective Review Panel
Toronto, CANADA

For additional copies please write or call:

PUBLICATIONS ONTARIO
50 Grosvenor St.
Toronto, Ontario M7A 1N8

Telephone: (416)-326-5300 or toll-free in Ontario 1-800-668-9938
Fax: (416)-326-5317
Hearing impaired call: (416)965-5130 or toll-free in Ontario 1-800-268-7095

Mastercard and Visa accepted. Cheques and money orders payable to the Minister of Finance. Prepayments required.

ISBN 0-7778-6242-5   Cat. #2228212   60M/04/97

Comment sheets are provided at the end of the document for the reader's suggestions.

While great effort has been taken to assure the accuracy of the information, the Review Panel, publisher, printer and others contributing to the preparation of this document cannot accept liability for errors, omissions or any consequences arising from the use of the information. Since this document is not intended to replace other prescribing information, physicians are urged to consult the manufacturer's and other available drug information literature before prescribing.

Acknowledgment: The production and distribution of this document was made possible through funding provided by the Ontario Ministry of Health.

TABLE OF CONTENTS

Respiratory Infections

Skin Infections

Genitourinary Infections

Central Nervous System Infections

Gastrointestinal Infections

Prophylaxis

Appendices

THE ANTI-INFECTIVE REVIEW PANEL
The panel represents a mix of health professionals with expertise in several fields, and who practise in a variety of clinical settings. Their names, areas of expertise and places of practice are listed below.

The panel was chaired by **Dr. Walter Rosser**, Professor and Chair, Department of Family and Community Medicine, Faculty of Medicine, University of Toronto.

Dr. Carolyn Bennett
Family Medicine
Toronto, Ontario

Dr. Andrew Braude
Respiratory/Internal
Medicine
North York General
Hospital
Willowdale, Ontario

Dr. Charles Chan
Respiratory/Internal
Medicine
Toronto Hospital
Toronto, Ontario

Dr. Gerald Evans
Infectious Diseases
Kingston General Hospital
Kingston, Ontario

Dr. Geordie Fallis
Family Medicine
Flemingdon Health Centre,
North York, Ontario

Dr. David Greenberg
Family Medicine
Toronto, Ontario

Dr. Barbara Liu
Geriatrics/Clinical
Pharmacology
Sunnybrook Health Science
Centre
Toronto, Ontario

Dr. Lionel Mandell
Infectious Diseases
McMaster Medical Unit/
Henderson General Hospital
Hamilton, Ontario

Dr. Ross Pennie
Pediatrics/Infectious
Diseases
Chedoke-McMaster
Hospitals
Hamilton, Ontario

Dr. Ross Prince
Urology
Oakville, Ontario

Dr. Colin Ramsay
Dermatology
Toronto, Ontario

Dr. Harold Richardson
Medical Microbiology
Chedoke-McMaster
Hospitals
Hamilton, Ontario

Dr. John Rutka
ENT
The Toronto Hospitals
Toronto, Ontario

Dr. John Stewart
Family Medicine
Port Perry, Ontario

Dr. Irene Turpie
Geriatrics
St. Joseph's Community
Health Centre
Hamilton, Ontario

Deanne Wong
Drug Information Specialist
Ontario College of
Pharmacists
Toronto, Ontario

GUIDELINE REVIEWERS

Many thanks to the individuals below who painstakingly reviewed the first and second edition of the guidelines and provided numerous suggestions to help improve the document. We look forward to your continued support.

Dr. Neal Stein
Family Medicine
Ajax, Ontario

Dr. M.J. Stephenson
Dr. Peggy Barringer
Family Medicine
Ancaster, Ontario

Dr. Peter Dalziel
Dr. Wendy Lambert
Family Medicine
Barrie, Ontario

Dr. Ian Maxwell
Emergency Medicine
Barrie, Ontario

Leo N. Fortin
Pharmacy
Belleville, Ontario

Dr. I.G. Cowan
Family Medicine
Borden, Ontario

Dr. Paul Hoy
Family Medicine
Bowmanville, Ontario

Dr. Thomas Klein
Ophthalmology
Brampton, Ontario

Dr. E. Waitschies
Dr. Wayne McShane
Family Medicine
Brampton, Ontario

Dr. Tae Bin Toby Im
Family Medicine
Brantford, Ontario

Dr. Gerald P. Ashe
Family Medicine
Brockville, Ontario

Dr. William Love Jr.
Urology
Burlington, Ontario

Dr. Dennis Brodie
Emergency Medicine
Burlington, Ontario

Dr. Robert Henderson
Family Medicine
Cambellford, Ontario

Dr. John B. Erb
Family Medicine
Cambridge, Ontario

Dr. Dave Lenny
Family Medicine
Carleton Place, Ontario

Dr. Caroline A. Knight
Family Medicine
Chesley, Ontario

Dr. Maurice O'Neil
Emergency Medicine
Collingwood, Ontario

Bill Wilson
Pharmacy
Copper Cliff, Ontario

Dr. John Joanisse
Family Medicine/Geriatrics,
Cumberland, Ontario

Dr. N. R. Flett
Family Medicine/Geriatrics
Dundas, Ontario

Dr. Kanwal Shankardass
Family Medicine
Dundas, Ontario

Dr. Keith W. Mabee
Family Medicine
Gananoque, Ontario

Dr. Milton Po
Radiation Oncology
Gloucester, Ontario

Dr. Sheila McCrae
Family Medicine
Gore Bay, Ontario

Dr. C. Parker
Dr. Peter Vaughan
Family Medicine
Guelph, Ontario

Dr. Nick Doroszkiewicz
Family Medicine
Hagersville, Ontario

Dr. Robert Heyes
Dr. Karl Hartwick
Family Medicine
Haliburton, Ontario

Margaret Wing
Pharmacy
Haliburton, Ontario

Hamilton
Dr. Mitchell Levine
Internal Medicine and
Clinical Pharmacology

Dr. Brian Haynes
Internal Medicine and
Epidemiology

Dr. Michael Rachlis
Internal Medicine/Geriatrics

Dr. H. Hotz
Pediatrics

Dr. C.E. Evans
Family Medicine/Surgery

Dr. Coleman Rotstein
Dr. Fiona Smaill
Infectious Diseases

Dr. A. Holbrook
Clinical Pharmacology

Dr. Tim Hillson
Dr. Michael J. Pray
Dr. W.R. Bullock
Dr. Philip Yanover
Dr. Ross Parker
Dr. J. Mullens
Family Medicine

Dr. Grant Seifred
Emergency Medicine

Patrick Wong
Pharmacy
Hawkesbury, Ontario

Dr. Lynn M. Fischer
Dr. Julie Bihun
Family Medicine
Kanata, Ontario

Kingston
Dr. John O'Quinn
Dr. Peter S. MacDonald
Internal Medicine

Dr. G.I. Stewart
Dr. R Schwartz
Dr. Sally Sharpe
Dr. John A. Geddes
Dr. Rupa Patel
Dr. Ian Crawford
Dr. P.G. Hodgetts
Family Medicine

Dr. Curtis Nickel
Urology

Dr. F.W. Danby
Dermatology

John McBride
Pharmacy

Dr. Mary Jackson
Respiratory Medicine
Kitchener, Ontario

A.D. Gulak
Pharmacy
Kitchener, Ontario

Dr. Roy Collins
Pharmacy
Lombardy, Ontario

London
Dr. D.B. Gregson
Infectious Diseases

Dr. Amin Murji
Dr. Gary Neumann
Dr. Barbara Lent
Dr. G.L Dickie
Family Medicine

Dr. Mary Mattar
Pediatrics

Dr. M. Forse
Respiratory Medicine
Markham, Ontario

Dr. Merilyn McTavish
Family Medicine
Midland, Ontario

Dr. Simon Brown
Dr. L. Grbac
Family Medicine
Mississauga, Ontario

Nepean
George A. O'Donnell
Pharmacy

Dr. Elaine Scales
Dr. Karen Hall
Family Medicine

Dr. Gordon Wallace
Emergency Medicine

Dr. D.M. Clark
Family Medicine
North Bay, Ontario

Oakville
Robert L. Green
Pharmacy

Dr. Janette White
Ophthalmology

Dr. Grahame Owen
Family Medicine

Anne Mallin
Pharmacy
Orangeville, Ontario

Dr. John W. Toye
Plastic Surgery
Orillia, Ontario

Dr. Tony Reid
Family Medicine
Orillia, Ontario

Dr. R. Lewans
Family Medicine
Orleans, Ontario

Ottawa
Dr. Nora MacDonald
Infectious Diseases/Pediatrics

Claudia McKeen
Pharmacy

Dr. Douglas Andrew Cochen
Resident OB/GYN

Dr. R. Hodder
Respiratory Medicine

Dr. Paul Gully
STD Control

Dr. J.E. Adam
Dermatology

Dr. Aaron Bernstein
Dr. R. Kelly McGinnis
Dr. D.J. Hilborn
Dr. Daniel Way
Dr. A. Donohue
Dr. Peter Teitelbaum
Dr. Christie MacDonald
Family Medicine

Dr. Marianne Yeung
Emergency Medicine

Dr. D.J. Stern
Family Medicine
Parry Sound, Ontario

Dr. G.W. Powell
Family Medicine
Peterborough, Ontario

Vern Chiles
Pharmacy
Sarnia, Ontario

Dr. James I. Leeson
Family Medicine
Sauble Beach, Ontario

Dr. Robert Maloney
Family Medicine/Emergency
Sault Ste. Marie, Ontario

Dr. Rasendra P. Kashyap
Dr. Edward Chow
Family Medicine
Scarborough, Ontario

Dr. Stewart Harris
Family Medicine
Sioux Lookout, Ontario

Dr. Karen Breeck
Family Medicine
Smooth Rock Falls, Ontario

Dr. Tim Prince
Family Medicine
St. Catharines, Ontario

Dr. Cathy Faulds
Family Medicine
St. Thomas, Ontario

Dr. J.N. Marshall
Family Medicine
Strathroy, Ontario

Dr. A. van Walraven
Internal Medicine
Stratford, Ontario

Dr. Mark A. Wilkinson
Family Medicine
Stratford, Ontario

Dr. Richard Payton
Family Medicine
Sudbury, Ontario

Dr. David A. Apramian
Family Medicine
Sundridge, Ontario

Dr. Henry H. Chapeskie
Family Medicine
Thorndale, Ontario

Dr. Arlen Rosenberg
Family Medicine
Thornhill, Ontario

Dr. Lawrence A. Lewis
Dr. Stephen Roedde
Emergency Medicine
Thunder Bay, Ontario

Dr. C. Cannon
Dr. Paul Humphries
Family Medicine
Thunder Bay, Ontario

Dr. Gaylen Kelton
Family Medicine/Emergency
Timmins, Ontario

Dr. M.V. Ciccone
Emergency Medicine
Timmins, Ontario

Toronto
Dr. George Y. Hiraki
General Surgery

Dr. S. Epstein
Internal Medicine

Dr. William Watson
Family Medicine/Emergency

Dr. Philip Berger,
Family Medicine and HIV/AIDS

Dr. Gerald I. Goldlist
Ophthalmology

Dr. N. Colodny
Dr. Peter D. Hopkins
Dr. W. Rubenstein
Dr. A. Cahalan
Dr. Susan Rosenthal
Dr. Marion C. Jewell
Dr. David W. Grossman
Dr. A.S. Geffen
Dr. David Smith
Dr. Sonny Cejic
Dr. Sonal Dholakie
Dr. Patricia Wilson-Jones
Family Medicine

Dr. William Feldman
Dr. J. Carlson,
Pediatrics

Dr. Anita Rachlis
Infectious Diseases

Dr. Pilon
Emergency Medicine

Dr. S.D. Abrahamson
Dr. J. Rieger
Anaesthesia and
Intensive Care Unit

Dr. Michael Hawke
Otolaryngology

Dr. Jay Keystone
Internal Medicine and
Travel Medicine

Dr. Andrew McIvor
Dr. Ronald Grossman
Respiratory Medicine

Mitra Montazari
Steven Schachter
Adrianna Hordienko
Fred J. Hearn
Lane Ilersich
Kalyna Butler
Shelley Diamond
Pharmacy

Dr. Andrew Simor
Infect Diseases and
Medical Microbiology

Dr. D.E. Low
Medical Microbiology

Dr. John M. Conly
Infectious Diseases and
Internal Medicine

Dr. Neil Shear
Dermatology

Denise Gelinas
Pharmacy
Vanier, Ontario

Dr. Ruth Hill
Family Medicine
Vanier, Ontario

Dr. Michel Blondin
Family Medicine
Vankleek Hill, Ontario

Dr. R.N. Libman
Family Medicine
Weston, Ontario

Louise L. Smith
Pharmacy
Whitby, Ontario

Dr. Ronald H. Smuckler
Dr. N.L. Sischly
Family Medicine
Willowdale, Ontario

Dr. Bill Bastianon
Family Medicine
Windsor, Ontario

Out of Province
Alberta
Dr. Pieter Oosthuisen
Family Medicine

Rob Moore
Pharmacy

Dr. Allen Ausford
Family Medicine

Dr. Stephen Shafran
Infectious Diseases

British Columbia
Dr. D.J. Natha
Dr. Tracy Monk
Dr. Kay Ho
Dr. Peter Battershell
Dr. Paul Chabun
Dr. Gerd A. Asche
Dr. C. Addison
Dr. E. John Booth
Dr. Todd Loewen
Dr. Mark Bigham
Dr. Brandt Miles
Dr. Marianne Rev
Dr. Stephen S. H. Ng
Dr. Louis Wilson
Dr. Mary-Stewart Moore
Dr. C. Gerbis
Dr. S.R. Long
Dr. Bob Henderson
Family Medicine

Dr. D. Scheifle
Infectious Diseases/Pediatrics

Dr. R. Tan
Medical Microbiology

Janet Webb
Pharmacy

Dr. Roy John Oakey
Emergency Medicine

Karen Dennis
Pharmacy

Manitoba
Dr. Lindsey Nicolle
Infectious Diseases

Dr. Antonio J. Sevilla
Family Medicine

George G. Zhavel
Pharmacy

North West Territories
Dr. Adele Dyall
Family Medicine

Nova Scotia
Dr. Mel Lee
Family Medicine

Quebec
Dr. Maryse Desmarais
Emergency Medicine

Dr. Jack Mendelsohn
Infectious Diseases and
Medical Microbiology

Dr. Jean Dzineku
Family Medicine and
Infections and Pediatrics

Isabelle Toillon
Pharmacy

Dr. Neil K. Hilliard
Family Medicine

Saskatchewan
Julie Campbell
Pharmacy

Dr. Leon A. Hart
Family Medicine

Paul Melnyk
Pharmacy

International
Dr. Chris Ross
Emergency Medicine
Chicago, Illinois

Dr. Allen Boettcher
Family Medicine
Atwood, Kansas

Dr. Jesus Juan Rodriguez
Infectious Diseases
Pinar Del Rio, Cuba

PROFESSIONAL ASSOCIATIONS & INDUSTRY

Ontario Hospital Association
Ontario Medical Association
Ontario Pharmacists' Association

College of Physicians and Surgeons of Ontario
Lyme Disease Association of Ontario
Pharmaceutical Manufacturers (25 companies)

PREFACE

Two years have passed since the release of the first edition of the guidelines and we have received many positive comments regarding its content and user-friendliness. In hindsight we can confidently say that it was well worth the extra time that it took to survey the needs of family practitioners regarding content and format.

The introduction of many new anti-infectives in the past 10 years has made it difficult for family physicians to know the specific role of each of these agents in the treatment of infectious diseases. To make their job easier, the Ontario Anti-infective Review Panel, an independent body composed of family physicians, specialists and pharmacists, has developed general guidelines.

Physicians generally base therapeutic decisions on their clinical experience, specific patient factors, laboratory results, available medical information plus advice from colleagues and experts. These guidelines are intended to meet the needs of family physicians for concise, relevant advice when initially selecting antimicrobial therapy for common community infections.

The panel believes these guidelines, which are updated regularly with the latest information on anti-infectives and feedback from physicians, can be a complementary, educational tool to promote the most appropriate use of medications and the best practice of medicine. However, they are not intended to replace a physician's judgment.

The development process of the first edition of these guidelines included a review of existing Canadian and international guidelines on the use of anti-infectives, including recommendations from seven major Canadian guidelines. From this knowledge base the panel produced draft guidelines that were discussed at four consensus conferences attended by family physicians, specialists and pharmacists. The meetings were also attended by representatives of the Canadian Drug Manufacturers Association, Canadian Society of Hospital Pharmacists, Ontario Pharmacists' Association, Pharmaceutical Manufacturers Association of Canada and the Ontario Ministry of Health.

The panel then sought feedback from 120 medical practitioners (general and specialists) and associations across Canada. Their recommendations were reviewed, without revealing their identity to the panel, at a fifth consensus conference and many were used in the final text.

The production of reputable, clinical guidelines is a continual process requiring the active, ongoing participation of physicians. The panel produced the second edition of the guidelines after reviewing all comments that were submitted after the publishing of the first edition. Based on these comments and availability of scientific literature several changes were made and new sections added.

The panel strongly encourages you to send your suggestions and recommendations on the comment page at the back of the booklet. They will all be thoroughly reviewed prior to publication of the third edition. We look forward to receiving your continuing support and participation.

USE OF THE GUIDELINES

General
Selecting the appropriate antibiotic involves consideration of the location of the infection and clinical diagnosis, sensitivity patterns of possible organisms involved, host factors, treatment setting and cost (when efficacy and toxicity issues are equivalent). Where possible the committee has made an effort to provide specific drug choices, rather than broad classes, since this is more practical and useful to family physicians.

The first, second and third line choices of antibiotics in these guidelines have been carefully selected based on spectrum of activity, anticipated efficacy, safety, previous clinical experience and resistance patterns. Many of the second and third line agents are often as effective as first line agents. They have been made alternatives because of important considerations such as intolerance, spectrum of activity, potential noncompliance, and cost. In general, the older antibiotics should not be discarded for newer drugs unless efficacy is substantially improved, toxicity is reduced, or overall cost effectiveness is greater.

Dosage/Dosage Form
An effort has been made to suggest oral products, wherever feasible and the products listed can be assumed to be for oral consumption unless designated otherwise. In the geriatric population, intravenous (IV) antibiotics should be avoided where possible, since IV therapy often involves immobilizing the frail elderly. The panel has attempted to ensure that the dosage suggestions are in accord with accepted standards, however physicians are advised to consult the product monograph and other sources for additional information on age and condition specific dosing. This is particularly important with new or infrequently used drugs.

Prices/Costs
An approximate daily treatment cost for adults has been included for each anti-infective agent. For children, a cost per kilogram per day (cost/kg/day) is estimated from available oral liquid preparations or solid dosage forms. Prices used for determining daily costs were derived initially from the Ontario Drug Benefit Formulary (35th edition) and if no listing was found the manufacturers' price lists were consulted. It is acknowledged that acquisition price will vary according to individual pharmacy practices and thus the estimated daily costs may not reflect all community situations. **The daily cost does not include a dispensing fee or markup.**

ACKNOWLEDGMENTS

We wish to acknowledge the assistance and expertise offered by physicians, pharmacists and manufacturers throughout the process, and those individuals who reviewed the draft of the document and provided invaluable input. A special note of appreciation is due to Dr. Walter Rosser, Professor & Chair, Department of Family and Community Medicine, University of Toronto, who offered excellent consensus facilitation to the panel, and to Medication Use Management Services (M.U.M.S.) Inc. for preparation of the background conference materials and the final document.

Respiratory Infections

Modifying Circumstances	Probable Organism(s)		Antibiotic Choice(s)	Usual Dosage‡	Cost per day*

Pharyngitis [1]

Modifying Circumstances	Probable Organism(s)		Antibiotic Choice(s)	Usual Dosage‡	Cost per day*
ADULT	**VIRAL**		**No antibiotics indicated**		
	BACTERIAL Strep Group A	*FIRST LINE*	Penicillin V	300mg (500,000 units) TID or 600mg BID	$0.12- $0.16
		SECOND LINE	Erythromycin	1g/day divided BID TID or QID	$0.21- $1.50
		THIRD LINE	Cephalexin	250mg QID	$0.69
			Clarithromycin	250mg BID	$2.96
			Azithromycin [2]	500mg for 1 day then 250mg daily x 4 days	5 day treatment: $29.60
CHILDREN [3]	**VIRAL**		**No antibiotics indicated**		
	BACTERIAL Strep Group A	*FIRST LINE*	Penicillin V	25-50mg/kg/day divided q6-8h	$0.02- $0.04/kg
			Amoxicillin	40mg/kg/day divided q8h	$0.03/kg
			Pivampicillin	40-60mg/kg/day divided q12h	$0.07- $0.11/kg
		SECOND LINE	Erythromycin estolate	30-40mg/kg/day divided q6-8h	$0.03- $0.04/kg
		THIRD LINE	Cephalexin	25-50mg/kg/day divided q6h	$0.04- $0.07/kg

1) Note that approximately 80 - 90% of the time pharyngitis is not bacterial in adults or children. Criteria for bacterial infection in adults are **absence of cough, history of fever over 38°C (101°F), tonsillar exudate**, and **swollen, tender anterior nodes**. If only one of the four clinical findings are present, then neither a throat swab nor antibiotics are indicated. If two or three criteria are present a throat culture is recommended and antibiotics started only if culture is positive. Antibiotic therapy can be delayed by 48-72 hours without increased risk of rheumatic fever. If all 4 criteria are present penicillin may be considered immediately based on clinical grounds (Centor, 1981).

2) Azithromycin has a long half-life (69 hrs) and requires only a single 5 day course of treatment.

3) Criteria for bacterial infection in children include **fever > 39.5°C , pharyngeal exudate, tender submandibular lymph nodes and palatine stippling**. A child who presents with three criteria has an 83% positive predictive value for streptococcal throat infection and this increases to 88% if four criteria are met. If less than three criteria are met then it is likely to be viral or a lower respiratory infection (Breese et al., 1985).

©1997 Ontario's Anti-infective Guidelines: TMP/SMX=Trimethoprim/Sulfamethoxazole

‡ Common oral dosage ranges are provided unless otherwise stated. Consult the drug monogragh for details on age and condition specific dosing.

* Approximate costs were derived from the ODB formulary (# 35) or manufacturers' price lists and do not include professional fees or markups.   *Page 2*

Modifying Circumstances	Probable Organism(s)	Antibiotic Choice(s)	Usual Dosage[‡]	Cost per day*

Epiglottitis - *MEDICAL EMERGENCY* [1,2]

Modifying Circumstances	Probable Organism(s)		Antibiotic Choice(s)	Usual Dosage[‡]	Cost per day*
ADULT & CHILDREN	H. influenzae type B	*FIRST LINE*	**Cefuroxime IV** [3]	750-1500mg q8h	$25.00-$50.34
				Children: 200mg/kg/day divided q8h (max: 4.5g/day)	$2.13/kg
PRIORITY IS TO ESTABLISH AIRWAY CONTROL			**Cefotaxime IV**	1-2g q8h	$27.60- $55.20
				Children: 100-150 mg/kg/day divided q6-8h	$0.93- $1.38/kg
			Ceftriaxone IV	1-2g q24h	$34.00- $67.00
				Children: 50-100 mg/kg/day divided q24h	$1.70- $3.40/kg
		SECOND LINE	**Chloramphenicol IV**	50-100mg/kg/day divided q6h	1g vial: $3.73
				Children: 75-100mg/kg/day divided q6h	$0.28- $0.37/kg

1) Adults are also at risk of contracting this disease. This infection has almost completely disappeared in children due to immunization against H. influenzae B. If epiglottitis is suspected, one should also consider bacterial tracheitis.

2) Ampicillin should be used when cultures demonstrate sensitive organisms.

3) Some children undergoing treatment for epiglottitis have subsequently developed meningitis. Therefore, a higher dose of cefuroxime is recommended in case there is unrecognized meningitis.

©1997 Ontario's Anti-infective Guidelines: TMP/SMX=Trimethoprim/Sulfamethoxazole

‡ Common oral dosage ranges are provided unless otherwise stated. Consult the drug monogragh for details on age and condition specific dosing.
* Approximate costs were derived from the ODB formulary (# 35) or manufacturers' price lists and do not include professional fees or markups.   *Page 3*

Modifying Circumstances	Probable Organism(s)	Antibiotic Choice(s)	Usual Dosage‡	Cost per day*

Laryngitis [1]

Modifying Circumstances	Probable Organism(s)	Antibiotic Choice(s)	Usual Dosage‡	Cost per day*
INCLUDES LARYNGO-TRACHEO-BRONCHITIS OR CROUP	Viral	No antibiotic indicated		

1) Bacterial tracheitis and epiglottitis should be ruled out because these require antibiotic therapy.

Acute Rhinitis (Common Cold)

Modifying Circumstances	Probable Organism(s)	Antibiotic Choice(s)	Usual Dosage‡	Cost per day*
	Viral	No antibiotic indicated		

‡ Common oral dosage ranges are provided unless otherwise stated. Consult the drug monogragh for details on age and condition specific dosing.
* Approximate costs were derived from the ODB formulary (# 35) or manufacturers' price lists and do not include professional fees or markups. *Page 4*

Modifying Circumstances	Probable Organism(s)		Antibiotic Choice(s)	Usual Dosage[‡]	Cost per day[*]

Otitis Externa *('Swimmer's Ear')* - *Acute and Uncomplicated* [1,2]

Modifying Circumstances	Probable Organism(s)		Antibiotic Choice(s)	Usual Dosage	Cost per day
ADULT & CHILDREN	Coliforms S. aureus Ps. aeruginosa	FIRST LINE	SOFRACORT [3] otic solution	Instill 2 to 3 drops TID or QID	8mL bottle: $10.40
			GARASONE [4] otic solution	Instill 3 to 4 drops TID	7.5mL bottle: $12.82
			BURO-SOL [5] otic solution	Instill 2 to 3 drops TID or QID	15mL bottle: $2.45
		SECOND LINE	CORTISPORIN [6] otic solution	Instill 4 drops TID or QID Children: Instill 3 drops TID or QID.	7mL bottle: $8.05

1) **PROPHYLAXIS:** A few drops of vinegar in the ear each time after swimming is a reasonable preventative strategy.

INFECTION ONLY: A steroid is useful where there is an underlying dermatitis. If it appears to be purely an infection an aminoglycoside product without a steroid can be used. If it persists after 7 days then re-assess, consider referral.

2) If TYMPANIC PERFORATION is present note that pain is usually experienced when drops reach the middle ear through the perforated membrane. This is a result of the acid and alcohol content of the otic preparation. An ophthalmic preparation (e.g. CORTISPORIN®) may have less acid. In the presence of a tympanic membrane perforation the risk of ototoxicity with topical aminoglycosides may increase when duration of therapy extends beyond seven days. Refer to specialist if condition does not settle.

3) SOFRACORT® contains 5mg framycetin sulfate, 0.05mg of gramicidin and 0.5mg dexamethasone per mL.

4) GARASONE® contains 3mg of gentamicin sulfate and 1mg of betamethasone sodium phosphate per mL.

5) BURO-SOL® contains 0.5% aluminum acetate and 0.03% benzethonium chloride in a dilute acetic acid solution.

OTORRHEA: A topical antiseptic (BURO-SOL®) rather than a topical antibiotic should be considered for the initial treatment of otorrhea on the grounds of cost, avoidance of resistance and toxicity. The clinical efficacy was assessed of a topical antiseptic (aluminum acetate) and a topical antibiotic (gentamicin) for initial treatment of otorrhea. No significant difference was found between the 2 treatment groups (68% resolution with gentamicin versus 67% with antiseptic). No resistant organisms to aluminum acetate were encountered, whereas 12 gentamicin treated cases had gentamicin resistant organisms at presentation and 1 patient developed a gentamicin resistant pseudomonas. (Clayton et al., 1990)

6) CORTISPORIN® contains 10,000 U polymyxin sulfate, 5mg neomycin sulfate and 10mg hydrocortisone per mL.

©1997 Ontario's Anti-infective Guidelines: TMP/SMX=Trimethoprim/Sulfamethoxazole

[‡] Common oral dosage ranges are provided unless otherwise stated. Consult the drug monogragh for details on age and condition specific dosing.
[*] Approximate costs were derived from the ODB formulary (# 35) or manufacturers' price lists and do not include professional fees or markups.   *Page 5*

Modifying Circumstances	Probable Organism(s)		Antibiotic Choice(s)	Usual Dosage‡	Cost per day*

Otitis Externa -Adult: Acute complicated (soft tissue infection)

Modifying Circumstances	Probable Organism(s)		Antibiotic Choice(s)	Usual Dosage‡	Cost per day*
MILD TO MODERATE	Coliforms S. aureus	*FIRST LINE*	TMP/SMX	2 tabs BID or 1 DS tab BID	$0.33
	Ps. aeruginosa[1]		**Cloxacillin**	250-500mg QID	$0.40- $0.78
			Cephalexin	250mg QID	$0.69
			Amoxicillin/Clavulanate	250mg TID	$2.62
SEVERE [2,3,4]	Ps. aeruginosa	*FIRST LINE*	**Ciprofloxacin**	500-750mg BID	$5.01- $9.45
		SECOND LINE	**Gentamicin IV** [5] OR	4 to 6mg/kg q24h	80mg vial: $4.17
			Tobramycin IV [5] OR	4 to 6mg/kg q24h	80mg vial: $6.89
			Amikacin IV [5]	15-20mg/kg q24h	500mg vial: $29.25
			PLUS ONE OF FOLLOWING		
			Ticarcillin IV	3g q3-6h	$50.04- $100.08
			Piperacillin IV	3-4g q4-6h	$75.60- $126.00
			Ciprofloxacin IV	400mg q12h	$66.00
			Imipenem IV	500mg q6h	$98.68
			Ceftazidime IV	2g q8h	$111.30

1) Note that Ps. aeruginosa is not a tissue invader in an otherwise normal host.
2) Includes individuals with malignant otitis externa, diabetes mellitus and/or who are immunocompromised.
3) Treat from four to eight weeks; local treatment with topical antibiotic drops usually required concomitantly.
4) If hospitalized, initiate treatment with double coverage, once patient stabilizes discontinue the aminoglycoside. When clinical conditions allow consider oral ciprofloxacin.
5) Gentamicin, tobramycin and amikacin may be given q24h rather than the conventional dosing of q8h for short term use where there is normal creatinine clearance. If duration of therapy extends beyond 2 or 3 days check creatinine clearance. With continued use beyond 5 days increased surveillance is recommended due to the potential for nephrotoxicity and ototoxicity, especially in elderly patients (ototoxicity manifests either with dizziness/imbalance or hearing loss initially, depending on the aminoglycoside). For more information see page 90 or consider consulting a specialist.

©1997 Ontario's Anti-infective Guidelines: TMP/SMX=Trimethoprim/Sulfamethoxazole

‡ Common oral dosage ranges are provided unless otherwise stated. Consult the drug monogragh for details on age and condition specific dosing.
* Approximate costs were derived from the ODB formulary (# 35) or manufacturers' price lists and do not include professional fees or markups.   *Page 6*

Modifying Circumstances	Probable Organism(s)		Antibiotic Choice(s)	Usual Dosage‡	Cost per day*

Otitis Externa -Children: Acute complicated (soft tissue infection)

Modifying Circumstances	Probable Organism(s)		Antibiotic Choice(s)	Usual Dosage‡	Cost per day*
MILD TO MODERATE	Coliforms S. aureus	*FIRST LINE*	TMP/SMX	8-12mg/kg/day divided q12h	$0.02-$0.03/kg
	Ps. aeruginosa[1]		Cloxacillin	50-100mg/kg/day divided q6h	$0.05-$0.10/kg
			Cephalexin	25-50mg/kg/day divided q6h	$0.04-$0.07/kg
			Amoxicillin/Clavulanate	40mg/kg/day amoxicillin divided q8h	$0.15/kg
SEVERE		*FIRST LINE*	Hospital admission for IV therapy		

1) Note that Ps. aeruginosa is not a tissue invader in an otherwise normal host.

Modifying Circumstances	Probable Organism(s)		Antibiotic Choice(s)	Usual Dosage‡	Cost per day*

Otitis Externa - Otomycosis [1,2]

Modifying Circumstances	Probable Organism(s)		Antibiotic Choice(s)	Usual Dosage‡	Cost per day*
ADULT & CHILDREN	FUNGAL Candida albicans	FIRST LINE	Clotrimazole 1% cream	Apply BID (am and hs)	30g: $3.42
	Aspergillus niger		Tolnaftate 1% cream	Apply BID (am and hs)	15g: $3.55
			LOCACORTEN-VIOFORM drops [3]	Instill 2 to 3 drops BID	10mL: $12.30

1) If recurrent, may require a referral to a specialist. Rule out diabetes if recurrent.
2) If no response is seen with tolnaftate or clotrimazole cream, consider aspergillus niger as a possible cause and treat with an agent that will cover (i.e. itraconazole). Consider referral to specialist.
3) LOCACORTEN-VIOFORM®: Each 10mL contains flumethasone pivalate 0.02% and clioquinol 1.0%.

Otitis Externa - Furuncle or Pustule

Modifying Circumstances	Probable Organism(s)	Antibiotic Choice(s)	Usual Dosage‡	Cost per day*
ADULT AND CHILDREN	S. aureus	Refer to Cutaneous Abscesses in Skin Infection Section		

©1997 Ontario's Anti-infective Guidelines: TMP/SMX=Trimethoprim/Sulfamethoxazole

‡ Common oral dosage ranges are provided unless otherwise stated. Consult the drug monogragh for details on age and condition specific dosing.
* Approximate costs were derived from the ODB formulary (# 35) or manufacturers' price lists and do not include professional fees or markups.   **Page 8**

Modifying Circumstances	Probable Organism(s)		Antibiotic Choice(s)	Usual Dosage‡	Cost per day*

Otitis Media - Adult: Acute

Modifying Circumstances	Probable Organism(s)		Antibiotic Choice(s)	Usual Dosage‡	Cost per day*
WITH OR WITHOUT PERFORATION	S. pneumoniae H. influenzae	*FIRST LINE*	**Amoxicillin**	250-500mg TID	$0.31- $0.60
	M. catarrhalis Strep. Group A	*SECOND LINE*	**TMP/SMX**	2 tabs BID or 1 DS tab BID	$0.33
	S. aureus		**Pivampicillin**	500mg BID	$1.32
	Gram -ve bacilli		**Amoxicillin/Clavulanate**	250-500mg TID	$2.62 - $4.08
	Anaerobes		**Doxycycline**	100mg BID first day then 100mg daily	$1.70
	Respiratory viruses		**Cefaclor**	250-500mg BID-TID	$1.53 - $4.50
			Cefuroxime-AX	250mg BID	$2.89
			Cefprozil	250mg BID	$3.00
			Cefixime	400mg daily	$3.09
			Clarithromycin	250-500mg BID	$2.96- $5.92
			Azithromycin [1]	500mg first day then 250mg daily x 4 days	5 day treatment: $29.60
PROPHYLAXIS [2]	Same as above	*FIRST LINE*	**TMP/SMX** **Amoxicillin** **Pivampicillin**	The literature is unclear on the most effective dosage.	

1) Azithromycin has a long half-life (69 hrs) and requires only a single 5 day course of treatment.
2) These guidelines do not address the controversy of whether medical or surgical therapy is optimal for recurrent attacks of otitis media with effusion persisting more than 12 weeks.

©1997 Ontario's Anti-infective Guidelines: TMP/SMX=Trimethoprim/Sulfamethoxazole

‡ Common oral dosage ranges are provided unless otherwise stated. Consult the drug monogragh for details on age and condition specific dosing.
* Approximate costs were derived from the ODB formulary (# 35) or manufacturers' price lists and do not include professional fees or markups. ***Page 9***

Modifying Circumstances	Probable Organism(s)		Antibiotic Choice(s)	Usual Dosage[‡]	Cost per day[*]

Otitis Media - Children: Acute [1]

Modifying Circumstances	Probable Organism(s)		Antibiotic Choice(s)	Usual Dosage[‡]	Cost per day[*]
WITH OR WITHOUT PERFORATION	S. pneumoniae	FIRST LINE	Amoxicillin	40mg/kg/day divided q8h	$0.03/kg
	H. influenzae		TMP/SMX	8-12mg/kg/day trimethoprim divided q12h	$0.02- $0.03/kg
	M. catarrhalis	SECOND LINE	Pivampicillin	40-60mg/kg/day divided q12h	$0.07- $0.11/kg
			Amoxicillin/Clavulanate	40mg/kg/day amoxicillin divided q8h	$0.15/kg
			Cefixime	8mg/kg/day divided q12-24h	$0.13/kg
			Cefaclor [3]	40mg/kg/day divided q8-12h	$0.17/kg
			Cefprozil	30mg/kg/day divided q12h	$0.18/kg
			Cefuroxime-AX	30-40mg/kg/day divided q12h	$0.18 - $0.26/kg
			ER/SX [2]	40mg/kg/day erythromycin divided q6-8h	$0.10/kg
			Clarithromycin	15mg/kg/day divided q12h	$0.16/kg
			Azithromycin [4]	10mg/kg on day one then 5mg/kg days 2 - 5	5 day treatment: $1.34/kg
PROPHYLAXIS [5]	Same as above	FIRST LINE	TMP/SMX Amoxicillin Pivampicillin	Prophylactic dose for children is one half usual therapeutic dose BID	

1) Antimicrobial drugs have a modest but significant impact on the primary control of acute otitis media. Treatment with ß-lactamase-stable agents does not increase resolution of acute symptoms or middle ear effusion; initial therapy should be guided by considerations of safety, tolerability, and affordability, and not by the theoretical advantage of an extended antibacterial spectrum. A meta-analysis of 5400 children from 33 randomized trials found spontaneous resolution (without antibiotics or tympanocentesis) occurred in 81% of cases. Compared with placebo or no drug, antimicrobial therapy increased resolution by 13.7%. No differences were found in the comparative efficacy of various antimicrobial agents (Rosenfeld et al., 1994).
2) ER/SX is Erythromycin ethylsuccinate/Sulfisoxazole. Erythromycin alone is not recommended because it does not cover H. influenzae adequately.
3) Infrequent cases of a serum sickness-like reaction (reported at 0.024% in overall clinical trials) have been associated with cefaclor but have caused little sustained morbidity. The relative risk is, however, greater with cefaclor than with amoxicillin and penicillin V. This reaction is more likely to occur in children under the age of six years who have had multiple courses, during the winter months and with the liquid preparation.
4) Azithromycin has a long half-life (69 hrs) and requires only a single 5 day course of treatment.
5) When symptoms persist a concurrent viral infection often appears to be responsible; when infection recurs the pathogen is often a new bacterial strain (Arola et al., 1990; Del Beccaro et al., 1992). These guidelines do not address the controversy of whether medical or surgical therapy is optimal for recurrent attacks of otitis media with effusion persisting more than 12 weeks.

©1997 Ontario's Anti-infective Guidelines: TMP/SMX=Trimethoprim/Sulfamethoxazole

‡ Common oral dosage ranges are provided unless otherwise stated. Consult the drug monogragh for details on age and condition specific dosing.
* Approximate costs were derived from the ODB formulary (# 35) or manufacturers' price lists and do not include professional fees or markups.   *Page 10*

Modifying Circumstances	Probable Organism(s)		Antibiotic Choice(s)	Usual Dosage‡	Cost per day*

Otitis Media - Chronic Suppurative [1,2]

Modifying Circumstances	Probable Organism(s)		Antibiotic Choice(s)	Usual Dosage‡	Cost per day*
ADULT & CHILDREN PERFORATION OR CHOLESTEA-TOMA	Polymicrobial S. aureus Proteus sp. Klebsiella E. coli B. fragilis	FIRST LINE	Mild cases may be treated topically with: SOFRACORT [3] otic solution GARASONE [4] otic solution	 Instill 2 to 3 drops TID or QID Instill 3 to 4 drops TID	 8mL bottle: $10.40 7.5mL bottle: $12.82
	Ps. aeruginosa	SECOND LINE	CORTISPORIN [5] otic solution Systemic antibiotics for significant soft tissue infection: TMP/SMX	Instill 4 drops TID or QID Children: Instill 3 drops TID or QID 2 tabs BID or 1 DS tab BID Children: 8-12mg/kg/day trimethoprim divided q12h	7mL bottle: $8.05 $0.33 $0.02- $0.03/kg
			Cephalexin	250mg QID Children: 25-50mg/kg/day divided q6h	$0.69 $0.04- $0.07/kg
			Amoxicillin/Clavulanate	250mg TID Children: 40mg/kg/day amoxicillin divided q8h	$2.62 $0.15/kg

1) Treatment with antibiotics alone (topical or parenteral) is rarely successful unless there is careful cleaning of the external canal and frequent microdebridements as often as necessary to keep canal clean and dry. If no response, consider treating with an antibiotic that covers Ps. aeruginosa. May require surgical (mastoidectomy) treatment for cholesteatoma or recalcitrant cases. Referral to ENT specialist may be necessary.

2) The risk of ototoxicity with topical aminoglycoside increases with duration of therapy beyond seven days.

3) SOFRACORT® contains 5mg framycetin sulfate, 0.05mg of gramicidin and 0.5mg dexamethasone per mL.

4) GARASONE® contains 3mg of gentamicin sulfate and 1mg of betamethasone sodium phosphate per mL.

5) CORTISPORIN® contains 10,000 U polymyxin sulfate, 5mg neomycin sulfate and 10mg hydrocortisone per mL.

©1997 Ontario's Anti-infective Guidelines: TMP/SMX=Trimethoprim/Sulfamethoxazole

‡ Common oral dosage ranges are provided unless otherwise stated. Consult the drug monogragh for details on age and condition specific dosing.
* Approximate costs were derived from the ODB formulary (# 35) or manufacturers' price lists and do not include professional fees or markups.   Page 11

Modifying Circumstances	Probable Organism(s)		Antibiotic Choice(s)	Usual Dosage[‡]	Cost per day*

Sinusitis - Adult: *Acute* [1,2,3,4]

Modifying Circumstances	Probable Organism(s)		Antibiotic Choice(s)	Usual Dosage[‡]	Cost per day*
	S. pneumoniae	**FIRST LINE**	**Amoxicillin**	500mg TID	$0.60
	H. influenzae				
	M. catarrhalis		**TMP/SMX**	2 tabs BID or 1 DS tab BID	$0.33
	Strep. Group A				
	S. aureus	**SECOND LINE**	**Pivampicillin**	500mg BID	$1.32
	Gram -ve bacilli		**Amoxicillin/Clavulanate**	500mg TID	$4.08
	Anaerobes		**Doxycycline**	100mg BID first day then 100mg daily	$1.70
	Respiratory viruses		**Cefuroxime-AX**	250mg BID	$2.89
			Cefaclor	500mg BID-TID	$3.00 - $4.50
			Cefprozil	250-500mg BID	$3.00 - $6.00
			Cefixime	400mg daily	$3.09
			Clarithromycin	250-500mg BID	$2.96- $5.92
			Azithromycin [5]	500mg first day then 250mg daily x 4 days	5 day treatment: $29.60

1) Considered in combination, maxillary toothache, poor response to nasal decongestants, coloured nasal discharge by history or examination and abnormal transillumination are the most useful indicators of sinusitis. When none of these is present sinusitis is virtually ruled out. Other symptoms that may increase the likelihood of sinusitis include fever, malaise, cough, and headache or facial pain exacerbated by bending forward. Sinus aspiration and culture is appropriate for guiding antibiotic choice in complicated or refractory sinusitis. (Williams, 1993)

2) Duration of therapy has generally been 10 to 14 days. One study suggests that for afebrile patients who are not immunocompromised, a 3 day course of TMP/SMX plus a nasal decongestant (e.g. oxymetazoline) can be prescribed. The patient should be counselled to expect symptoms to disappear within 14 days. (Williams, 1995)

3) Saline rinses may be beneficial.

4) For recurrent or chronic sinusitis exclude the possibility of anatomical abnormalities which may require surgery. In chronic sinusitis antimicrobials do not usually play a major role.

5) Azithromycin has a long half-life (69 hrs) and requires only a single 5 day course of treatment.

©1997 Ontario's Anti-infective Guidelines: TMP/SMX=Trimethoprim/Sulfamethoxazole

‡ Common oral dosage ranges are provided unless otherwise stated. Consult the drug monogragh for details on age and condition specific dosing.
* Approximate costs were derived from the ODB formulary (# 35) or manufacturers' price lists and do not include professional fees or markups.   *Page 12*

Modifying Circumstances	Probable Organism(s)		Antibiotic Choice(s)	Usual Dosage‡	Cost per day*

Sinusitis - Children: Acute [1,2,3]

Modifying Circumstances	Probable Organism(s)		Antibiotic Choice(s)	Usual Dosage‡	Cost per day*
	S. pneumoniae H. influenzae	**FIRST LINE**	**Amoxicillin**	40mg/kg/day divided q8h	$0.03/kg
	M. catarrhalis Strep.Group A	**SECOND LINE**	**TMP/SMX**	8-12mg/kg/day trimethoprim divided q12h	$0.02- $0.03/kg
	S. aureus		**Pivampicillin**	40-60mg/kg/day divided q12h	$0.07- $0.11/kg
	Gram -ve bacilli		**Amoxicillin/Clavulanate**	40mg/kg/day amoxicillin divided q8h	$0.15/kg
	Anaerobes Respiratory viruses		**Cefixime**	8mg/kg/day divided q12-24h	$0.13/kg
			Cefaclor [5]	40mg/kg/day divided q8-12h	$0.17/kg
			Cefprozil	15-30mg/kg/day divided q12h	$0.09-$0.18/kg
			Cefuroxime-AX	30-40mg/kg/day divided q12h	$0.18-$0.26/kg
			ER/SX [4]	40mg/kg/day erythromycin divided q6-8h	$0.10/kg
			Clarithromycin	15mg/kg/day divided q12h	$0.16/kg
			Azithromycin [6]	10mg/kg on day one, then 5mg/kg days 2 - 5	5 day treatment: $1.34/kg

1) The sinuses become fully developed in children between the age of five and seven years. Consider acute sinusitis in children of five years of age and over. For recurrent or chronic sinusitis exclude the possibility of anatomical abnormalities which may require surgery.

2) Two common features - persistent symptoms and severe symptoms - may suggest the child has acute sinusitis. Persistent symptoms are those that last more than 10 days and less than 30 days and have not begun to improve. The 10 day mark differentiates simple viral infection from sinusitis and the 30 day mark separates acute from subacute or chronic sinusitis.
Symptoms of sinusitis: Nasal discharge (may be thin or thick and clear mucoid or purulent), daytime cough and may worsen at night. The child may not appear very ill and with low grade fever. Sinusitis may also present as an unusually severe upper respiratory infection with severe symptoms (high fever, purulent nasal discharge). (Wald, 1992)

3) Safety is very important when treating a condition with an approximate 40% spontaneous cure rate. Hence amoxicillin is acceptable and preferred for most uncomplicated cases of sinusitis. Duration of therapy has not been well studied. Empirically a 10 - 14 day course of therapy is recommended. (Wald, 1992)

4) ER/SX is erythromycin ethylsuccinate/sulfisoxazole. Erythromycin alone is not recommended because it does not cover H. influenzae adequately.

5) Infrequent cases of a serum sickness-like reaction (reported at 0.024% in overall clinical trials) have been associated with cefaclor but have caused little sustained morbidity. The relative risk is, however, greater with cefaclor than with amoxicillin and penicillin V. This reaction is more likely to occur in children under the age of six years who have had multiple courses, during the winter months and with the liquid preparation.

6) Azithromycin has a long half-life (69 hrs) and requires only a single 5 day course of treatment.

©1997 Ontario's Anti-infective Guidelines: TMP/SMX=Trimethoprim/Sulfamethoxazole

‡ Common oral dosage ranges are provided unless otherwise stated. Consult the drug monograph for details on age and condition specific dosing.
* Approximate costs were derived from the ODB formulary (# 35) or manufacturers' price lists and do not include professional fees or markups. **Page 13**

Modifying Circumstances	Probable Organism(s)		Antibiotic Choice(s)	Usual Dosage‡	Cost per day*

Acute Bronchitis: Adults [1]

Modifying Circumstances	Probable Organism(s)		Antibiotic Choice(s)	Usual Dosage‡	Cost per day*
MILD TO SEVERE	**VIRAL**		**No antibiotic indicated**		
	BACTERIAL Mycoplasma pneumonia S. pneumonia C. pneumonia	*FIRST LINE*	Tetracycline	250mg QID	$0.08
			Erythromycin	1g/day divided BID TID or QID	$0.21- $1.50
		SECOND LINE	Doxycycline [2]	100mg BID first day then 100mg daily	$1.70
			Clarithromycin	250-500mg BID	$2.96- $5.92
			Azithromycin [3]	500mg first day then 250mg daily x 4 days	5 day treatment: $29.60

1) 80% of all cases of acute bronchitis are viral, however, it is difficult to reliably distinguish between these etiologies since both viral and bacterial pathogens may result in purulent sputum (Boldy et al., 1990). Onset of productive cough and wheezing are the most common symptoms. An evaluation of the current literature does not support routine antibiotic treatment for acute bronchitis (Orr, 1993). **Primary prevention must be emphasized, such as the reduction of risk factors (e.g., smoking).**
2) There is limited evidence that doxycycline may have small beneficial effects in patients with acute cough and purulent sputum (Verheij, 1994). These beneficial effects are more prominent in patients age 55 years and over.
3) Azithromycin has a long half-life (69 hrs) and requires only a single 5 day course of treatment.

Acute Bronchitis: Children

	VIRAL [1]	*FIRST LINE*	**No antibiotic indicated**		

1) (Chapman, 1981)

©1997 Ontario's Anti-infective Guidelines: TMP/SMX=Trimethoprim/Sulfamethoxazole

‡ Common oral dosage ranges are provided unless otherwise stated. Consult the drug monogragh for details on age and condition specific dosing.
* Approximate costs were derived from the ODB formulary (# 35) or manufacturers' price lists and do not include professional fees or markups. **Page 14**

Modifying Circumstances	Probable Organism(s)		Antibiotic Choice(s)	Usual Dosage‡	Cost per day*

Acute Exacerbations of Chronic Bronchitis - Adult
Mild to moderate clinical presentation [1,2]

Modifying Circumstances	Probable Organism(s)		Antibiotic Choice(s)	Usual Dosage‡	Cost per day*
LIMITED UNDERLYING LUNG DISEASE	S. pneumoniae H. influenzae Moraxella catarrhalis Mycoplasma pneumoniae	*FIRST LINE*	Tetracycline	250mg QID	$0.08
			TMP/SMX	2 tabs BID or 1 DS tab BID	$0.33
			Amoxicillin	500mg TID	$0.62
		SECOND LINE	Doxycycline	100mg BID first day then 100mg daily	$1.70
			Amoxicillin/Clavulanate	250-500mg TID	$2.62- $4.08
			Cefaclor	250-500mg TID	$2.30 -$4.50
			Cefuroxime-AX	250mg BID	$2.89
			Clarithromycin	250-500mg BID	$2.96- $5.92
			Azithromycin [3]	500mg first day then 250mg daily x 4 days	5 day treatment: $29.60

1) Adapted from Forward et al., 1990 Consensus recommendations for management of acute exacerbations of chronic bronchitis and Balter et al., 1994 Recommendations on the Management of Chronic Bronchitis.
2) Fifty percent of A.E.C.B. are non-bacterial. Chronic bronchitis is defined clinically as excessive cough, productive of sputum on most days, for at least 3 months a year during at least two consecutive years. Diagnosis is based on a history of increased cough or sputum production, increased sputum purulence and increased dyspnea. Cigarette smoking is the most common cause of chronic bronchitis and cessation produces dramatic symptomatic benefits. The use of antimicrobials to treat A.E.C.B. is the most contentious aspect of the management of this disease.
3) Azithromycin has a long half-life (69 hrs) and requires only a single 5 day course of treatment.

©1997 Ontario's Anti-infective Guidelines: TMP/SMX=Trimethoprim/Sulfamethoxazole

‡ Common oral dosage ranges are provided unless otherwise stated. Consult the drug monogragh for details on age and condition specific dosing.
* Approximate costs were derived from the ODB formulary (# 35) or manufacturers' price lists and do not include professional fees or markups.   *Page 15*

Modifying Circumstances	Probable Organism(s)		Antibiotic Choice(s)	Usual Dosage‡	Cost per day*

Acute Exacerbations of Chronic Bronchitis - Adult
Severe clinical presentation [1,2]

Modifying Circumstances	Probable Organism(s)		Antibiotic Choice(s)	Usual Dosage‡	Cost per day*
EXTENSIVE UNDERLYING LUNG DISEASE and/or OTHER RISK FACTORS [3]	S. pneumoniae H. influenzae Moraxella catarrhalis Mycoplasma pneumoniae	FIRST LINE	TMP/SMX	2 tabs BID or 1 DS tab BID	$0.33
			Amoxicillin/Clavulanate	500mg TID	$4.08
			Cefaclor	250-500mg TID	$2.30 - $4.50
			Cefuroxime-AX	250mg- 500mg BID	$2.89-$5.73
			ANY ONE of the above +/- Erythromycin [4]	1g/day divided BID TID or QID	$0.21- $1.50
			Clarithromycin [4]	250-500mg BID	$2.96- $5.92
			Azithromycin [4,5]	500mg first day then 250mg daily x 4 days	5 day treatment: $29.60
		SECOND LINE	Ofloxacin	400mg BID	$4.86
			Ciprofloxacin	500-750mg BID	$5.01- $9.45

1) Fifty percent of A.E.C.B. are non-bacterial. Chronic bronchitis is defined clinically as excessive cough, production of sputum on most days, for at least 3 months a year during at least two consecutive years. Cigarette smoking is the most common cause of chronic bronchitis and cessation produces dramatic symptomatic benefits. (Balter et al., 1994 Recommendations on the Management of Chronic Bronchitis).

2) For IV options see severe pneumonia.

3) Risk factors may include: poor pulmonary function (FEV, below 50% of predicted level), age over 65 years, comorbid medical illness (congestive heart failure, diabetes, chronic renal failure, chronic liver disease).

4) Erythromycin **must** be used in conjunction with one of the other four agents because it does not have consistently reliable activity against H. influenzae.
If clarithromycin or azithromycin is used, they may be used alone.

5) Azithromycin has a long half-life (69 hrs) and requires only a single 5 day course of treatment.

©1997 Ontario's Anti-infective Guidelines: TMP/SMX=Trimethoprim/Sulfamethoxazole

‡ Common oral dosage ranges are provided unless otherwise stated. Consult the drug monogragh for details on age and condition specific dosing.
* Approximate costs were derived from the ODB formulary (# 35) or manufacturers' price lists and do not include professional fees or markups.   Page 16

Modifying Circumstances	Probable Organism(s)	Antibiotic Choice(s)	Usual Dosage‡	Cost per day*

Bronchiectasis: *Acute Infective Exacerbations* [1,2,3]

Modifying Circumstances	Probable Organism(s)	Antibiotic Choice(s)	Usual Dosage‡	Cost per day*
	H. influenzae **FIRST** S. pneumoniae **LINE** Moraxella catarrhalis	**TMP/SMX**	2 tabs BID or 1 DS tab BID Children: 8-12mg/kg/day trimethoprim q12h	$0.33 $0.02- $0.03/kg
		Amoxicillin/Clavulanate	500mg TID Children: 40mg/kg/day amoxicillin divided q8h	$4.08 $0.15/kg
	Ps. aeruginosa	**Ciprofloxacin**	500-750mg BID Children: Not approved. Special cases exist. 20-30mg/kg/day q12h	$5.01- $9.45 $0.13 - $0.20/kg

1) For suppression of symptoms, long term low dose antibiotic therapy may be required for several months. Fluoroquinolones (ciprofloxacin) should not be used in this instance, as resistance may build up quickly.
2) Antimicrobial therapy should be directed by cultures.
3) The most common cause of bronchiectasis in children is cystic fibrosis. A cystic fibrosis patient should not be managed by a family practitioner in isolation; consultation with a specialist is recommended.

©1997 Ontario's Anti-infective Guidelines: TMP/SMX=Trimethoprim/Sulfamethoxazole

‡ Common oral dosage ranges are provided unless otherwise stated. Consult the drug monogragh for details on age and condition specific dosing.
* Approximate costs were derived from the ODB formulary (# 35) or manufacturers' price lists and do not include professional fees or markups. **Page 17**

Modifying Circumstances	Probable Organism(s)		Antibiotic Choice(s)	Usual Dosage‡	Cost per day*

Pneumonia – Adult, Community-acquired, mild to moderate [1]

Modifying Circumstances	Probable Organism(s)		Antibiotic Choice(s)	Usual Dosage‡	Cost per day*
NO COMORBIDITY [2]	S. pneumoniae Mycoplasma pneumoniae	*FIRST LINE*	Tetracycline [3]	250mg QID	$0.08
			Erythromycin	1g/day divided BID, TID or QID	$0.21- $1.50
	Chlamydia pneumoniae	*SECOND LINE*	Doxycycline [3]	100mg BID first day then 100mg daily	$1.70
	H. influenzae		Clarithromycin	250-500mg BID	$2.96- $5.92
			Azithromycin [4]	500mg first day then 250mg x 4 days	5 day treatment: $29.60
COMORBIDITY PRESENT [2]	Mixed infection: S. pneumoniae	*FIRST LINE*	TMP/SMX	2 tabs BID or 1 DS tab BID.	$0.33
	H. influenzae		Cefaclor	250mg TID	$2.30
	Oral anaerobes		Cefuroxime-AX	500mg BID	$5.73
	Gram -ve bacilli		Amoxicillin/Clavulanate	500mg TID	$4.08
	S. aureus				
	Legionella sp.		If Legionella sp. is a concern ANY ONE of the above PLUS: Erythromycin [5]	1g/day divided BID, TID or QID	$0.21- $1.50
			Clarithromycin [5]	250-500mg BID	$2.96- 5.92
			Azithromycin [4, 5]	500mg first day then 250mg x 4 days	5 day treatment: $29.60

1) This section was adapted from Mandell LA, Niederman M. The Canadian community acquired pneumonia consensus group. Antimicrobial treatment of community acquired pneumonia in adults, 1993. Note: The specific agents listed here may vary from the original document.
2) Comorbid illness includes but is not limited to COPD, diabetes mellitus, renal insufficiency, heart failure, or recent hospitalization within one year of the presentation with pneumonia.
3) Approximately 10% of pneumococci are resistant to tetracyclines.
4) Azithromycin has a long half-life (69 hrs) and requires only a single 5 day course of treatment.
5) A macrolide should be added if legionella is a concern. Erythromycin **must** be used in conjunction with one of the other four agents because it does not have consistently reliable activity against H. influenzae.
If clarithromycin or azithromycin is used, they may be used alone.

‡ Common oral dosage ranges are provided unless otherwise stated. Consult the drug monogragh for details on age and condition specific dosing.
* Approximate costs were derived from the ODB formulary (# 35) or manufacturers' price lists and do not include professional fees or markups.

Modifying Circumstances	Probable Organism(s)	Antibiotic Choice(s)	Usual Dosage[‡]	Cost per day[*]

Pneumonia -Adult, *Community-acquired, severe (in-hospital)*[1,2]

Modifying Circumstances	Probable Organism(s)		Antibiotic Choice(s)	Usual Dosage[‡]	Cost per day[*]
WITH OR WITHOUT COMORBIDITY [3]	S. pneumoniae H. influenzae	FIRST LINE	Cefuroxime-AX	500mg BID	$5.73
	Legionella sp.		Cefuroxime IV/IM	750mg -1.5g q8h	$23.51-$47.03
	Mycoplasma pneumoniae		Cefotaxime IV	1-2g q6-8h	$27.60- $73.60
	S. aureus		Ceftriaxone IV/IM	1-2g q24h or 500mg-1g q12h	$34.00 - $68.00
	C. pneumoniae				
	If comorbidity present other pathogens include: Oral anaerobes Gram -ve bacilli		ANY ONE of the above +/-		
			Erythromycin IV OR	500mg-1g q6h	$37.40-$55.40
			Clarithromycin OR	500mg BID	$5.92
			Azithromycin [4]	500mg first day then 250mg x 4 days	5 day treatment: $29.60
			+/- Rifampin [5]	600mg in a single daily dose	$2.46
		SECOND LINE	TMP/SMX IV PLUS	4-5mg/kg/day divided q6-12h	5ml ampul: $5.75
			Erythromycin IV	500mg -1g q6h	$37.40- $55.40

1) This section was adapted from Mandell LA, Niederman M. The Canadian community acquired pneumonia consensus group. Antimicrobial treatment of community acquired pneumonia in adults, 1993.

2) Criteria for **severe** pneumonia is any one of the following: respiratory failure (Pa O_2 <60 mmHg-with exception of patients with COPD who may be hypoxemic without pneumonia); respiratory rate more than 30 per minute; sepsis with evidence of end organ dysfunction; extrapulmonary septic complication; cavitation or involvement of more than one lobe on chest radiograph.

3) Comorbid illness includes but is not limited to COPD, diabetes mellitus, renal insufficiency, heart failure, or recent hospitalization within one year of the presentation with pneumonia

4) Azithromycin has a long half-life (69 hrs) and requires only a single 5 day course of treatment.

5) Rifampin may be added if Legionella is documented by (1. culture, 2. serology, 3. a positive DFA) as it offers a theoretical advantage in cases where there is severe legionnaires disease.

‡ Common oral dosage ranges are provided unless otherwise stated. Consult the drug monogragh for details on age and condition specific dosing.
* Approximate costs were derived from the ODB formulary (# 35) or manufacturers' price lists and do not include professional fees or markups. *Page 19*

Modifying Circumstances	Probable Organism(s)	Antibiotic Choice(s)	Usual Dosage[‡]	Cost per day[*]

Pneumonia -Adult,Community-acquired, severe (intensive care unit)[1,2]

Modifying Circumstances	Probable Organism(s)	Antibiotic Choice(s)	Usual Dosage[‡]	Cost per day[*]
WITH OR WITHOUT COMORBIDITY [3]	S. pneumoniae *FIRST LINE*	Erythromycin IV	500mg-1g q6h	$37.40- $55.40
	H. influenzae	+\-		
	Legionella sp.	Rifampin [4]	600mg in a single daily dose	$2.46
	Gram -ve bacilli			
	Ps. aeruginosa[5]	PLUS ONE of the following:		
	S. aureus [6]	Ciprofloxacin IV	400mg q12h	$66.00
	M. pneumonia	OR		
	C. pneumoniae	Imipenem IV	500mg q6h	$98.68
		OR		
		Ceftazidime IV	2g q8h	$111.30

1) This section was adapted from Mandell LA, Niederman M. The Canadian community acquired pneumonia consensus group. Antimicrobial treatment of community acquired pneumonia in adults, 1993.

2) Criteria for severe pneumonia is any one of the following: respiratory failure (Pa O2 <60 mmHg-with exception of patients with COPD who may be hypoxemic without pneumonia); respiratory rate more than 30 per minute; sepsis with evidence of end organ dysfunction: extra pulmonary septic complication; cavitation or involvement of more than one lobe on chest radiograph.

3) Comorbid illness includes but is not limited to COPD, diabetes mellitus, renal insufficiency, heart failure, or recent hospitalization within one year of the presentation with pneumonia.

4) Rifampin may be added if Legionella is documented by (1. culture, 2. serology, 3. a positive DFA) as it offers a theoretical advantage in cases where there is severe legionnaires disease.

5) Due to high mortality associated with Ps. aeruginosa, an aminoglycoside should be added for at least the first few days, whether one uses a third generation cephalosporin, imipenem or ciprofloxacin.

6) First line therapy for S. aureus is a penicillinase-resistant semisynthetic penicillin (e.g., cloxacillin). The regimens suggested here, while not optimal, would provide reasonable coverage until cultures and sensitivities are available, at which time therapy may be altered.

©1997 Ontario's Anti-infective Guidelines: TMP/SMX=Trimethoprim/Sulfamethoxazole

‡ Common oral dosage ranges are provided unless otherwise stated. Consult the drug monogragh for details on age and condition specific dosing.
* Approximate costs were derived from the ODB formulary (# 35) or manufacturers' price lists and do not include professional fees or markups.   **Page 20**

Modifying Circumstances	Probable Organism(s)	Antibiotic Choice(s)	Usual Dosage‡	Cost per day*

Pneumonia - Nursing home: *mild to moderate*

Modifying Circumstances	Probable Organism(s)	Antibiotic Choice(s)	Usual Dosage‡	Cost per day*
	S. pneumoniae **FIRST LINE** H. influenzae	TMP/SMX	2 tabs BID or 1 DS tab BID.	$0.33
	Oral anaerobes	**Cefaclor**	250mg TID	$2.30
	Gram -ve bacilli	**Cefuroxime-AX**	500mg BID	$5.73
	S. aureus Legionella sp.	**Amoxicillin/Clavulanate** [1]	500mg TID	$4.08
		ANY ONE of the above +/-		
		Erythromycin [2]	1g divided BID, TID or QID	$0.21-$1.50
		Clarithromycin [2]	250-500mg BID	$2.96- $5.92
		Azithromycin [2, 3]	500mg first day then 250mg daily x 4 days	5 day treatment: $29.60

1) Amoxicillin/Clavulanate should be used if there is clinically apparent aspiration or a concern with anaerobes.
2) A macrolide should be added if Legionella is a concern. Erythromycin **must** be used in conjunction with one of the other four agents because it does not have consistently reliable activity against H. influenzae. If clarithromycin or azithromycin is used, they may be used alone.
3) Azithromycin has a long half-life (69 hrs) and requires only a single 5 day course of treatment.

©1997 Ontario's Anti-infective Guidelines: TMP/SMX=Trimethoprim/Sulfamethoxazole

‡ Common oral dosage ranges are provided unless otherwise stated. Consult the drug monogragh for details on age and condition specific dosing.
* Approximate costs were derived from the ODB formulary (# 35) or manufacturers' price lists and do not include professional fees or markups.

Modifying Circumstances	Probable Organism(s)	Antibiotic Choice(s)	Usual Dosage‡	Cost per day*

Pneumonia - Nursing home: *Severe* [1]

Modifying Circumstances	Probable Organism(s)	Antibiotic Choice(s)	Usual Dosage‡	Cost per day*
	S. pneumoniae **FIRST LINE**	**Amoxicillin/Clavulanate**	500mg TID	$4.08
	H. influenzae			
	Oral anaerobes	**Cefaclor**	500mg TID	$4.50
	Gram -ve bacilli			
	S. aureus	**Cefuroxime-AX**	500mg BID	$5.73
		Ceftriaxone IV/IM **OR the following combination:**	1-2g q24h or 500mg-1g q12h	$34.00- $67.00
		Penicillin V **OR**	300mg TID	$0.12
		Amoxicillin **PLUS**	500mg TID	$0.60
		Ciprofloxacin	750mg BID	$9.45
	Legionella sp.	**If Legionella sp. is a concern ANY ONE of the above PLUS:** **Erythromycin** [2]	1g divided BID, TID or QID	$0.21-$1.50
		Clarithromycin [2]	500mg BID	$5.92
		Azithromycin [2, 3]	500mg first day then 250mg daily x 4 days	5 day treatment: $29.60
	SECOND LINE	**Ciprofloxacin** **PLUS**	750mg BID	$9.45
		Clindamycin	300mg QID	$6.21

1) Criteria for severe pneumonia is any one of the following: respiratory failure (Pa O_2 <60 mmHg-with exception of patients with COPD who may be hypoxemic without pneumonia); respiratory rate more than 30/minute; sepsis with evidence of end organ dysfunction: extrapulmonary septic complication; cavitation or involvement of more than one lobe on chest radiograph. (Mandell and Niederman, 1993)
2) A macrolide should be added if Legionella is a concern. Erythromycin **must** be used in conjunction with one of the other four agents because it does not have consistently reliable activity against H. influenzae. If clarithromycin or azithromycin is used, they may be used alone.
3) Azithromycin has a long half-life (69 hrs) and requires only a single 5 day course of treatment.

©1997 Ontario's Anti-infective Guidelines: TMP/SMX=Trimethoprim/Sulfamethoxazole

‡ Common oral dosage ranges are provided unless otherwise stated. Consult the drug monogragh for details on age and condition specific dosing.
* Approximate costs were derived from the ODB formulary (# 35) or manufacturers' price lists and do not include professional fees or markups. **Page 22**

Modifying Circumstances	Probable Organism(s)		Antibiotic Choice(s)	Usual Dosage‡	Cost per day*

Pneumonia with Cystic Fibrosis: Children [1]

	S. aureus	FIRST LINE	Gentamicin IV [2]	7-10mg/kg/day divided q8-24h	$0.36 - $0.52/kg
			OR		
			Tobramycin IV [2]	7-10mg/kg/day divided q8-24h	$0.85 - $1.21/kg
			OR		
			Amikacin IV [2]	15-22.5mg/kg/day divided q8-q24h	$0.88 - $1.36/kg
			PLUS ONE of the following:		
			Ciprofloxacin IV	Not approved for use <18 years: Special cases exist. 20-30 mg/kg/day divided q12h	$1.65- $2.48/kg
			Ticarcillin IV	300mg/kg/day divided q4-6h	$1.25/kg
			Piperacillin IV	300mg/kg/day divided q6h	$2.21/kg
			Imipenem IV	Children >3 months: 60-100mg/kg/day divided q6h	$3.06- $5.10/kg
			Ceftazidime IV	100-200mg/kg/day divided q8h	$1.89- $3.77/kg

1) A cystic fibrosis patient should not be managed by a family practitioner in isolation; consultation with a specialist is required.
2) Q24h dosing is suitable for children beyond the neonatal period. Gentamicin, tobramycin and amikacin may be given q24h rather than the conventional dosing of q8h for short term use where there is normal creatinine clearance. If duration of therapy extends beyond 2 or 3 days check creatinine clearance. With continued use beyond 5 days increased surveillance is recommended due to the potential for nephrotoxicity and ototoxicity, especially in elderly patients (ototoxicity manifests either with dizziness/imbalance or hearing loss initially, depending on the aminoglycoside). For more information see page 90 or consider consulting a specialist.

©1997 Ontario's Anti-infective Guidelines: TMP/SMX=Trimethoprim/Sulfamethoxazole

‡ Common oral dosage ranges are provided unless otherwise stated. Consult the drug monogragh for details on age and condition specific dosing.
* Approximate costs were derived from the ODB formulary (# 35) or manufacturers' price lists and do not include professional fees or markups. **Page 23**

Modifying Circumstances	Probable Organism(s)	Antibiotic Choice(s)	Usual Dosage‡	Cost per day*

Pneumonia with Cystic Fibrosis: Adults [1]

Modifying Circumstances	Probable Organism(s)	Antibiotic Choice(s)	Usual Dosage‡	Cost per day*
	Ps. aeruginosa **FIRST LINE**	Gentamicin IV [2]	4 to 6 mg/kg q24h	80mg vial: $4.17
		OR		
		Tobramycin IV [2] OR	4 to 6 mg/kg q24h	80mg vial: $6.89
		Amikacin IV [2]	15-20mg/kg q24h	500mg vial: $29.25
		PLUS ONE of the following:		
		Ciprofloxacin IV	400mg q12h	$66.00
		Ticarcillin IV	3g q3-6h	$50.04- $100.08
		Imipenem IV	500mg q6h	$98.68
		Ceftazidime IV	2g q8h	$111.30
		Piperacillin IV	3-4g q4-6h	$75.60- $126.00

1) A cystic fibrosis patient should not be managed by a family practitioner in isolation; consultation with a specialist is required.

2) Gentamicin, tobramycin and amikacin may be given q24h rather than the conventional dosing of q8h for short term use where there is normal creatinine clearance. If duration of therapy extends beyond 2 or 3 days check creatinine clearance. With continued use beyond 5 days increased surveillance is recommended due to the potential for nephrotoxicity and ototoxicity, especially in elderly patients (ototoxicity manifests either with dizziness/imbalance or hearing loss initially, depending on the aminoglycoside). For more information see page 90 or consider consulting a specialist.

©1997 Ontario's Anti-infective Guidelines: TMP/SMX=Trimethoprim/Sulfamethoxazole

‡ Common oral dosage ranges are provided unless otherwise stated. Consult the drug monogragh for details on age and condition specific dosing.
* Approximate costs were derived from the ODB formulary (# 35) or manufacturers' price lists and do not include professional fees or markups. **Page 24**

Modifying Circumstances	Probable Organism(s)		Antibiotic Choice(s)	Usual Dosage‡	Cost per day*

Pneumonia - Children, [1] *Community-acquired*

	VIRAL		**No antibiotics indicated**		
MILD TO MODERATE	**BACTERIAL** S. pneumoniae	***FIRST LINE***	**Amoxicillin**	40mg/kg/day divided q8h	$0.03/kg
	S. aureus Strep. Group A		**Erythromycin estolate**	30-40mg/kg/day divided q12h	$0.03- $0.04/kg
	Mycoplasma pneumoniae	***SECOND LINE***	**TMP/SMX**	8-12mg/kg/day trimethoprim divided q12h	$0.02- $0.03/kg
	H. influenzae		**Pivampicillin**	40-60mg/kg/day divided q12h	$0.07- $0.11/kg
			Amoxicillin/Clavulanate	40mg/kg/day amoxicillin divided q8h	$0.15/kg
			Cefixime	8mg/kg/day divided q12-24h	$0.13/kg
			Cefaclor	40mg/kg/day divided q8h	$0.17/kg
			Cefuroxime-AX	40mg/kg/day divided q12h	$0.26/kg
			ER/SX [2]	40mg/kg/day erythromycin divided q6-8h	$0.10/kg
			Clarithromycin	15mg/kg/day divided q12h	$0.16/kg
			Azithromycin [3]	10mg/kg on day one, then 5mg/kg days 2 - 5	5 day treatment: $1.34/kg
SEVERE	S. pneumoniae S. aureus	***FIRST LINE***	**Cefuroxime IV** +/-	100-150mg/kg/day divided q8h	$1.07- $1.61/kg
	Strep. Group A Mycoplasma pneumonia		**Erythromycin estolate** OR	30-40mg/kg/day divided q6h	$0.03- $0.04/kg
			Clarithromycin	15mg/kg/day divided q12h	$0.16/kg
	H.influenzae	***SECOND LINE***	**Chloramphenicol IV** +/-	50-75mg/kg/day divided q6h	$0.18-$0.28/kg
			Erythromycin estolate OR	30-40mg/kg/day divided q6h	$0.03- $0.04/kg
			Clarithromycin	15mg/kg/day divided q12h	$0.16/kg

1) Viruses are responsible for pneumonia in the majority of children under five years of age.
2) ER/SX is Erythromycin ethylsuccinate/Sulfisoxazole.
3) Azithromycin has a long half-life (69 hrs) and requires only a single 5 day course of treatment.

‡ Common oral dosage ranges are provided unless otherwise stated. Consult the drug monogragh for details on age and condition specific dosing.
* Approximate costs were derived from the ODB formulary (# 35) or manufacturers' price lists and do not include professional fees or markups. **Page 25**

Modifying Circumstances	Probable Organism(s)	Antibiotic Choice(s)		Usual Dosage‡	Cost per day*

Pertussis (*Whooping Cough*) [1,2,3]

Modifying Circumstances	Probable Organism(s)		Antibiotic Choice(s)	Usual Dosage‡	Cost per day*
ADULT AND CHILDREN	Bordetella pertussis	*FIRST LINE*	Erythromycin (for adult)	1g/day divided BID, TID or QID	$0.21- $1.50
			Erythromycin estolate (for children)	Children: 30-40mg/kg/day divided q6-8h	$0.03- $0.04/kg
		SECOND LINE	TMP/SMX	2 tabs BID or 1 DS tab BID	$0.33
				Children: 8-12mg/kg/day divided q12h	$0.02- $0.03/kg
		THIRD LINE	Tetracycline [4]	250mg QID	$0.08
				Children: 25-50mg/kg/day divided q6h	$0.02- $0.04/kg
			Amoxicillin	250-500mg TID	$0.31- $0.60
				Children: 40mg/kg/day divided q8h	$0.15/kg
			Ampicillin	250mg QID	$0.33
				Children: 50mg/kg/day divided q6h	$0.03/kg
			Clarithromycin	250 - 500mg BID	$2.96 - $5.92
				Children: 15mg/kg/day divided q12h	$0.16/kg
			Azithromycin [5]	500mg first day then 250mg x 4 days	5 day treatment: $29.60
				Children: 10mg/kg on day one then 5mg/kg days 2-5	5 day treatment: $1.34/kg

1) Pertussis should be suspected (and reported to the Medical Officer of Health) in individuals with any duration of paroxysmal cough, or cough with inspiratory whoop, or cough ending in apnea, vomiting or gagging for which there is no other known cause (Canada Communicable Disease Report, 1993).
2) The treating physician should consult with public health authorities and ensure that all household contacts of cases have their immunization updated and are offered chemoprophylaxis; same drug regimen as for active case - see above (Canada Communicable Disease Report, 1994).
3) Duration of therapy is usually 10 days. However, antibiotic therapy started three weeks after the onset of symptoms is of no benefit since the organism has already been spontaneously cleared from the nasopharynx.
4) Tetracyclines should not be used in children under nine years of age unless there are compelling reasons to do so (e.g. Rickettsial infections) (Canadian Pediatric Society, 1994).
5) Azithromycin has a long half-life (69 hrs) and requires only a single 5 day course of treatment.

‡ Common oral dosage ranges are provided unless otherwise stated. Consult the drug monogragh for details on age and condition specific dosing.
* Approximate costs were derived from the ODB formulary (# 35) or manufacturers' price lists and do not include professional fees or markups.

Skin Infections

Modifying Circumstances	Probable Organism(s)	Antibiotic Choice(s)	Usual Dosage[‡]	Cost per day[*]

Impetigo & Bullous Impetigo - Adult [1,2]

Modifying Circumstances	Probable Organism(s)		Antibiotic Choice(s)	Usual Dosage[‡]	Cost per day[*]
	Strep. Group A S. aureus	FIRST LINE	Topical therapy in less severe cases:		
			Mupirocin 2% [3] ung	Apply sparingly TID	15g: $7.44
			Fusidic Acid 2% [4] ung/cream	Apply sparingly TID-QID. If covered with occlusive dressing then daily or BID	15g: $8.43
			Systemic agents for more significant soft tissue infection:		
			Cloxacillin	250-500mg QID	7-10 days: $2.78-$7.78
			Cephalexin	250mg QID	7-10 days: $4.83- $6.90
		SECOND LINE	Erythromycin	1g/day divided BID, TID or QID	$0.21- $1.50
			Clarithromycin	250mg BID	$2.96
			Clindamycin	150-300mg QID	$3.10- $6.21

1) The majority of infections can be treated topically. Use topical therapy when infection is limited and localized (i.e. two to three small areas). Consider systemic therapy if infection is widespread, if patient is immunocompromised, has valvular heart disease, fever, constitutional symptoms suggesting bacteremia or has not improved from topical therapy within 24-48 hours. Outbreaks cannot be treated with topical therapy; consider performing cultures if complicated and/or during epidemics.

Recurrent impetigo: the most common underlying factor is S. aureus carriage in the anterior nares or perineum. Evaluate by culturing and if positive treat topically with mupirocin or fusidic acid 2-3 times daily, for 2-3 days. Another common cause of recurrent impetigo is secondary bacterial impetiginization of underlying dermatoses such as eczema or psoriasis. In these cases, the impetigo still needs therapy with antibacterials, but the underlying disease should be treated as well.

2) Bullous impetigo is due to S. aureus with production of epidermolytic toxin locally.

3) Mupirocin is available as an ointment only.

4) It is not necessary to remove the crusts before application of fusidic acid.

©1997 Ontario's Anti-infective Guidelines: TMP/SMX=Trimethoprim/Sulfamethoxazole

[‡] Common oral dosage ranges are provided unless otherwise stated. Consult the drug monogragh for details on age and condition specific dosing.
[*] Approximate costs were derived from the ODB formulary (# 35) or manufacturers' price lists and do not include professional fees or markups. **Page 28**

Modifying Circumstances	Probable Organism(s)	Antibiotic Choice(s)	Usual Dosage‡	Cost per day*

Impetigo & Bullous Impetigo - Children [1,2]

Modifying Circumstances	Probable Organism(s)	Antibiotic Choice(s)	Usual Dosage‡	Cost per day*
	Strep. Group A S. aureus	**FIRST LINE** Topical therapy in less severe cases:		
		Mupirocin 2% [3] **ung**	Apply sparingly TID	15g: $7.44
		Fusidic Acid 2% [4] **ung/cream**	Apply sparingly TID-QID. If covered with occlusive dressing then daily or BID	15g: $8.43
		Systemic antibiotics for significant soft tissue infection:		
		Cephalexin	25-50mg/kg/day divided q6h	$0.04- $0.07/kg
		SECOND LINE Erythromycin estolate	30-40mg/kg/day divided q6-8h	$0.03- $0.04/kg
		Clindamycin	10-30mg/kg/day divided q6h	$0.05-$0.15/kg
		THIRD LINE Flucloxacillin [5]	25-50mg/kg/day divided q6h	$0.13- $0.25/kg
		Cloxacillin	50-100mg/kg/day divided q6h	$0.05- $0.10/kg

1) The majority of infections can be treated topically. Use topical therapy when infection is limited and localized (i.e. two to three small areas). Consider systemic therapy if infection is widespread, if patient is immunocompromised, has valvular heart disease, fever, constitutional symptoms suggesting bacteremia or has not improved from topical therapy within 24-48 hours. Outbreaks cannot be treated with topical therapy; consider performing cultures if complicated and/or during epidemics.

Recurrent impetigo: the most common underlying factor is S. aureus carriage in the anterior nares or perineum. Evaluate by culturing and if positive treat topically with mupirocin or fusidic acid 2-3 times daily, for 2-3 days. Another common cause of recurrent impetigo is secondary bacterial impetiginization of underlying dermatoses such as eczema or psoriasis. In these cases, the impetigo still needs therapy with antibacterials, but the underlying disease should be treated as well.

2) Bullous impetigo is due to S. aureus with production of epidermolytic toxin locally.

3) Mupirocin is available as an ointment only.

4) It has not been shown necessary to remove the crusts before application of fusidic acid.

5) Flucloxacillin, though more expensive than cloxacillin, requires only one-half the dose of cloxacillin, has better absorption and a superior taste. It is recommended instead of cloxacillin where a liquid preparation is required. Cephalexin is well absorbed, has an acceptable taste, and is much less expensive than flucloxacillin.

©1997 Ontario's Anti-infective Guidelines: TMP/SMX=Trimethoprim/Sulfamethoxazole

‡ Common oral dosage ranges are provided unless otherwise stated. Consult the drug monogragh for details on age and condition specific dosing.
* Approximate costs were derived from the ODB formulary (# 35) or manufacturers' price lists and do not include professional fees or markups. **Page 29**

Modifying Circumstances	Probable Organism(s)		Antibiotic Choice(s)	Usual Dosage‡	Cost per day*

Cutaneous Abscesses: Uncomplicated

Modifying Circumstances	Probable Organism(s)		Antibiotic Choice(s)	Usual Dosage‡	Cost per day*
FOLLICULITIS [1] AND FURUNCLE [2] (BOIL)	S. aureus	FIRST LINE	Usually self limiting. Systemic therapy not generally required.		
		SECOND LINE	Topical therapy in less severe cases:		
			Mupirocin 2% [3] ung	Apply sparingly TID	15g: $7.44
			Fusidic Acid 2% [4] ung/ cream	Apply sparingly TID-QID, If covered with occlusive dressing then daily or BID	15g: $8.43
COMPLICATED CARBUNCLES [5]	S. aureus	FIRST LINE	Cloxacillin	250-500mg QID	$0.40- $0.78
			Cephalexin	250-500mg QID	$0.69- $1.38
		SECOND LINE	Clindamycin	150-300mg QID	$3.10 - $6.21
		THIRD LINE	Erythromycin	1g/day divided BID, TID or QID	$0.21- $1.50
			Clarithromycin	250-500mg BID	$2.96- $5.92

1) Folliculitis is usually associated with an infected hair follicle. When assessing folliculitis, one should try to determine whether it is infectious or not. Infectious folliculitis usually presents as bigger pustules (2-3mm) compared with pseudofolliculitis (1-2mm). There is more inflammation as manifested by a red halo and tenderness. The lesions tend to be clustered rather than scattered.

Infectious folliculitis: is most commonly caused by S. aureus. Gram negative folliculitis caused by Enterobacteriacea may uncommonly develop in acne patients on long term antibiotics. When mild and limited, may respond to drying measures. Local compresses are beneficial. If there is no improvement or the disease is extensive, topical antibacterial therapy should be used. Systemic therapy is generally not required unless the infection has progressed to the extent that it has become a carbuncle.

Pseudomonas folliculitis: develops in patients using hot-tubs contaminated with Pseudomonas aeruginosa. It has a predilection for the lower torso and the axillae.

Non-infectious folliculitis (or pseudofolliculitis): is inflammation of the hair follicle secondary to friction, irritation or occlusion. It is treated by removing the causative factor, i.e. friction or occlusion. Application of a topical drying agent such as aluminum chloride hexahydrate solution or a hydro-alcoholic solution is beneficial.

2) Furuncles (boils) are abscesses that start in a hair follicle; for small boils hot compresses are usually sufficient, while for larger ones drainage is necessary.

3) Mupirocin is available as an ointment only.

4) It has not been shown necessary to remove the crusts before application of fusidic acid.

5) Carbuncles are deeper and more extensive; drainage is necessary.

©1997 Ontario's Anti-infective Guidelines: TMP/SMX=Trimethoprim/Sulfamethoxazole

‡ Common oral dosage ranges are provided unless otherwise stated. Consult the drug monogragh for details on age and condition specific dosing.
* Approximate costs were derived from the ODB formulary (# 35) or manufacturers' price lists and do not include professional fees or markups.   *Page 30*

Modifying Circumstances	Probable Organism(s)		Antibiotic Choice(s)	Usual Dosage‡	Cost per day*

Cutaneous Abscesses: Complicated [1,2]

Modifying Circumstances	Probable Organism(s)		Antibiotic Choice(s)	Usual Dosage‡	Cost per day*
DECUBITUS ULCERS	Polymicrobial	FIRST LINE	Ciprofloxacin +/-	500-750mg BID	$5.01- $9.45
PERI-RECTAL AND PERI-ANAL ABSCESSES			Metronidazole [3]	500mg TID	$0.17
			OR		
			Clindamycin [3]	150-300mg QID	$3.10- $6.21
		SECOND LINE	Amoxicillin/Clavulanate [3]	250-500mg TID	$2.62- $4.08
			TMP/SMX [4] OR	2 tabs BID or 1 DS tab BID	$0.33
			Ceftriaxone IM/IV [5]	1-2g q24h or 500mg-1g q12h	$34.00- $67.00
			+/-		
			Metronidazole [3]	500mg TID	$0.17
			OR		
			Clindamycin [3]	150-300mg QID	$3.10- $6.21
		THIRD LINE	(Cloxacillin IV	250-500mg q4-6h	$1.63-$4.88
			OR		
			Cefazolin IV)	1-2g q8h	$12.36- $24.72
			PLUS		
			Metronidazole IV	500mg q8h	$42.63
			PLUS ONE of:		
			Gentamicin IV [6]	4 to 6mg/kg q24h	80mg: $4.17
			Tobramycin IV [6]	4 to 6mg/kg q24h	80mg: $6.89
			Amikacin IV [6]	15-20mg/kg q24h	500mg: $29.25

1) Prevention is the best therapy for decubitus ulcers and abscesses. Local care may be adequate if there is no evidence of systemic infection or extensive ulceration. Incision/surgical drainage, debride and add antibiotics where necessary.

2) Avoid topical therapy, usually a systemic broad spectrum antibiotic is required. Use vancomycin for serious infections, osteomyelitis, and/or for culture documented MRSA (methicillin resistant S. aureus).

3) If anaerobes are an issue then clindamycin or metronidazole should be added. This will depend on the location (i.e. coccygeal ulcers, diabetic ulcers), spectrum of pathogens and severity of infection. Amoxicillin/Clavulanate covers anaerobes and can be used alone.

4) TMP/SMX should not be used if Ps. aeruginosa is present.

5) Due to its long half life ceftriaxone should be used in emergency departments to avoid hospitalization.

6) Gentamicin, tobramycin and amikacin may be given q24h rather than the conventional dosing of q8h for short term use where there is normal creatinine clearance. If duration of therapy extends beyond 2 or 3 days check creatinine clearance. With continued use beyond 5 days increased surveillance is recommended due to the potential for nephrotoxicity and ototoxicity, especially in elderly patients (ototoxicity manifests either with dizziness/imbalance or hearing loss initially, depending on the aminoglycoside). For more information see page 90 or consider consulting a specialist.

©1997 Ontario's Anti-infective Guidelines: TMP/SMX=Trimethoprim/Sulfamethoxazole

‡ Common oral dosage ranges are provided unless otherwise stated. Consult the drug monogragh for details on age and condition specific dosing.
* Approximate costs were derived from the ODB formulary (# 35) or manufacturers' price lists and do not include professional fees or markups.   *Page 31*

Modifying Circumstances	Probable Organism(s)	Antibiotic Choice(s)		Usual Dosage‡	Cost per day*

Cellulitis - Uncomplicated: Mild

Modifying Circumstances	Probable Organism(s)		Antibiotic Choice(s)	Usual Dosage‡	Cost per day*
ADULT AND CHILDREN	S. aureus (Penicillinase producing) Strep. Group A	FIRST LINE	Cloxacillin	250-500mg QID	$0.40- $0.78
				Children: 50-100mg/kg/day divided q6h	$0.05- $0.10/kg
			Cephalexin	250-500mg QID	$0.69
				Children: 25-50mg/kg/day divided q6h	$0.04- $0.07/kg
			Penicillin V [1]	300mg TID or QID	$0.12- $0.16
				Children: 25-50mg/kg/day divided q6-8h	$0.02- $0.04/kg
			Amoxicillin [1]	250-500mg TID	$0.31- $0.60
				Children: 40mg/kg/day divided q8h	$0.03/kg
		SECOND LINE	Erythromycin (for adults)	1g/day divided BID, TID or QID	$0.21- $1.50
			Erythromycin estolate (for children)	Children: 30-40mg/kg/day divided q12h	$0.03- $0.04/kg
		THIRD LINE	Clarithromycin	250mg BID	$2.96
				Children: 15mg/kg/day divided q12h	$0.16/kg
			Clindamycin	150-300mg QID	$3.10- $6.21
				Children: 10-30mg/kg/day divided q6h	$0.07- $0.22/kg

1) If Strep. Group A is strongly suspected clinically (rapid extension, sharply defined erythema, small vesicles at the active margin) then penicillin V or amoxicillin may be given. If there is some doubt regarding the probable organism cloxacillin or cephalexin should be used.

©1997 Ontario's Anti-infective Guidelines: TMP/SMX=Trimethoprim/Sulfamethoxazole

‡ Common oral dosage ranges are provided unless otherwise stated. Consult the drug monogragh for details on age and condition specific dosing.
* Approximate costs were derived from the ODB formulary (# 35) or manufacturers' price lists and do not include professional fees or markups. **Page 32**

Modifying Circumstances	Probable Organism(s)	Antibiotic Choice(s)	Usual Dosage‡	Cost per day*

Cellulitis - Uncomplicated: *Severe*

Modifying Circumstances	Probable Organism(s)	Antibiotic Choice(s)	Usual Dosage‡	Cost per day*
ADULT AND CHILDREN NON-FACIAL		*FIRST LINE* **Cloxacillin IV**	250-500mg q4-6h Children: 100-150mg/kg/day divided q6h	$1.63-$4.88 $0.35- $0.53/kg
		Cefazolin IV	1-2g q8h Children: 50-100mg/kg/day divided q8h	$12.36- $24.72 $0.21-$0.41/kg
		SECOND LINE **Clindamycin PO/IV**	PO: 300mg QID IV: 600mg q8h Children: IV 25-40mg/kg/day divided q6-8h	PO: $6.21 IV: $39.20 $0.54- $0.87/kg

©1997 Ontario's Anti-infective Guidelines: TMP/SMX=Trimethoprim/Sulfamethoxazole

‡ Common oral dosage ranges are provided unless otherwise stated. Consult the drug monogragh for details on age and condition specific dosing.
* Approximate costs were derived from the ODB formulary (# 35) or manufacturers' price lists and do not include professional fees or markups.   *Page 33*

Modifying Circumstances	Probable Organism(s)		Antibiotic Choice(s)	Usual Dosage‡	Cost per day*

Cellulitis - Special Considerations: Complicated

Modifying Circumstances	Probable Organism(s)		Antibiotic Choice(s)	Usual Dosage‡	Cost per day*
FACIAL ERYSIPELAS	Strep. Group A (majority)	*FIRST LINE* [1]	Cefazolin IV	1g q8h	$12.36
ADULT	S. aureus	*SECOND LINE*	Vancomycin IV	500mg q6h or 1g q12h	$104.88
CHILDREN	Strep. Group A S. aureus	*FIRST LINE*	Cefuroxime IV	100 -150mg/kg/day divided q8h	$1.07- $1.61/kg
	H. influenzae	*SECOND LINE*	Amoxicillin/Clavulanate OR	40mg/kg/day amoxicillin divided q8h	$0.15/kg
			(Chloramphenicol IV [1] +/-	50-75mg/kg/day divided q6h	$0.18-$0.28/kg
			Cloxacillin IV)	50-100 mg/kg/day divided q6h	$0.05- $0.10/kg
DIABETIC FOOT [2] **ADULT MILD**	S. aureus Strep. Group A Strep. Group B Enterococci	*FIRST LINE*	TMP/SMX PLUS	2 tabs BID or 1 DS tab BID	$0.33
			Metronidazole	500mg TID	$0.17
	Mixed aerobic and anaerobic	*SECOND LINE*	Amoxicillin/Clavulanate OR	250mg TID	$2.62
			(TMP/SMX PLUS	2 tabs BID or 1 DS tab BID	$0.33
			Clindamycin)	150mg-300mg QID	$3.10- $6.21
		THIRD LINE	Clindamycin	150-300mg QID	$3.10- $6.21
			PLUS ONE of the FOLLOWING:		
			Ofloxacin	200mg BID	$4.14
			Ciprofloxacin [3]	500-750mg BID	$5.01- $9.45

1) If H. influenzae is suspected use chloramphenicol.
2) Cultures should be done in diabetic patients if the cellulitis is recurrent or associated with a long standing ulceration.
3) Consider using ciprofloxacin if pseudomonas is present.

‡ Common oral dosage ranges are provided unless otherwise stated. Consult the drug monogragh for details on age and condition specific dosing.
* Approximate costs were derived from the ODB formulary (# 35) or manufacturers' price lists and do not include professional fees or markups. **Page 34**

Modifying Circumstances	Probable Organism(s)	Antibiotic Choice(s)		Usual Dosage‡	Cost per day*

Cellulitis - Special Considerations: Complicated cont...[1]

Modifying Circumstances	Probable Organism(s)	Antibiotic Choice(s)		Usual Dosage‡	Cost per day*
DIABETIC FOOT ADULT SEVERE	S. aureus Strep. Group A Polymicrobial	FIRST LINE	Ciprofloxacin PO/IV +/-	PO: 750mg BID IV: 400mg q12h	PO: $9.45 IV: $66.00
			Metronidazole [1] OR	500mg TID	$0.17
			Clindamycin [1]	150-300mg QID	$3.10-$6.21
		SECOND LINE	Amoxicillin/Clavulanate [1]	250-500mg TID	$2.62-$4.08
			TMP/SMX [2] OR	2 tabs BID or 1 DS tab BID	$0.33
			Ceftriaxone IM/IV +/-	1-2g divided q12-24h	$34.00-$67.00
			Metronidazole [1] OR	500mg TID	$0.17
			Clindamycin [1]	150-300mg QID	$3.10-$6.21
		THIRD LINE	(Cloxacillin PO/ IV OR	PO: 250-500mg QID IV: 250-500mg q4-6h	PO:$0.40 -$0.78 IV: $1.63 -$4.88
			Cefazolin IV) PLUS	1-2g q8h	$12.36 - $24.72
			Metronidazole IV PLUS ONE of:	500mg q8h	$42.63
			Gentamicin IV [3]	4 to 6mg/kg q24h	80mg: $4.17
			Tobramycin IV [3]	4 to 6mg/kg q24h	80mg: $6.89
			Amikacin IV [3]	15-20mg/kg q24h	500mg: $29.25
INVASIVE STREP. GROUP A [4] TOXIC SHOCK-LIKE SYNDROME		FIRST LINE	Clindamycin IV PLUS	600mg q8h	$39.20
			(Cefazolin IV OR	1g q8h	$12.36
			Penicillin G IV)	300,000-20 million units/day	$0.53- $13.88
		SECOND LINE	Clindamycin IV	600mg q8h	$39.20
		THIRD LINE	Vancomycin IV	1g q12h	$104.90

1) Cultures should be taken. Consider admission to hospital. If anaerobes are an issue then clindamycin or metronidazole should be added. This will depend on the location, spectrum of pathogens and severity of infection. Amoxicillin/Clavulanate covers anaerobes and can be used alone.
2) TMP/SMX should not be used if Ps. aeruginosa is present.
3) Gentamicin, tobramycin and amikacin may be given q24h rather than the conventional dosing of q8h for short term use where there is normal creatinine clearance. If duration of therapy extends beyond 2 or 3 days check creatinine clearance. With continued use beyond 5 days increased surveillance is recommended due to the potential for nephrotoxicity and ototoxicity, especially in elderly patients (ototoxicity manifests either with dizziness/imbalance or hearing loss initially, depending on the aminoglycoside). See page 90.
4) Reportable to the Local Medical Officer of Health. Treat for a minimum of 10 days. Prophylaxis of close household contacts is recommended (e.g. cephalexin x 10 days). Resistance to clindamycin is still < 2%.

©1997 Ontario's Anti-infective Guidelines: TMP/SMX=Trimethoprim/Sulfamethoxazole

‡ Common oral dosage ranges are provided unless otherwise stated. Consult the drug monogragh for details on age and condition specific dosing.
* Approximate costs were derived from the ODB formulary (# 35) or manufacturers' price lists and do not include professional fees or markups.

Modifying Circumstances	Probable Organism(s)		Antibiotic Choice(s)	Usual Dosage[‡]	Cost per day*

Bites - *(For infected bites <u>NOT</u> for prophylaxis)* [1,2]

Modifying Circumstances	Probable Organism(s)		Antibiotic Choice(s)	Usual Dosage[‡]	Cost per day*
CAT	P. multocida S. aureus	FIRST LINE	Amoxicillin/Clavulanate	250-500mg TID	$2.62 - $4.08
				Children: 40mg/kg/day amoxicillin divided q8h	$0.15/kg
		SECOND LINE	Tetracycline [3]	250-500mg QID	$0.08-$0.16
				Children: 25-50mg/kg/day divided q6h	$0.02-$0.04/kg
			Doxycycline [3]	100mg BID first day then 100mg daily	$1.70
				Children: 2-4mg/kg/day q12h on first day then half dose q24h	$0.34 - $0.68/kg
		THIRD LINE	Erythromycin (for adults)	1g/day divided BID, TID or QID	$0.21- $1.50
			Erythromycin estolate (for children)	30-40mg/kg/day q6h	$0.03- $0.04/kg
			Clarithromycin	250mg BID	$2.96
				Children: 15mg/kg/day q12h	$0.16/kg
DOGS AND OTHER WILD ANIMALS	Viridans Strep P. multocida Bacteroides Fusobacter	FIRST LINE	Amoxicillin/Clavulanate	250-500mg TID	$2.62- $4.08
				Children: 40mg/kg/day amoxicillin divided q8h	$0.15/kg
	EF-4 DF-2 (C. canimorsus)	SECOND LINE	Tetracycline [3]	250mg QID	$0.08
				Children: 25-50 mg/kg/day divided q6h	$0.02 - $0.04/kg
SEVERE WOUNDS		FIRST LINE	Ticarcillin/ Clavulanate IV	3.1g q4-8h	$28.33- $57.66
				Children: 200-300mg/kg/day divided q4-6h	$0.62- $0.93/kg
			Ceftriaxone IM/IV	1-2 g q24h or 500mg-1g q12h	$34.00 - $67.00
				Children: 50-100mg/kg/day divided q12-24h	$1.70- $3.40/kg

1) Refer to the Canadian Immunization Guide for management of rabies. Report to local public health office if potentially exposed to rabies (i.e. wild or domestic animal bite). Prophylaxis with antibiotics is controversial.
2) All wounds should be thoroughly cleaned, irrigated and debrided. Ensure tetanus prophylaxis is up to date.
3) Tetracyclines should not be used in children under nine years of age unless there are compelling reasons to do so (e.g. Rickettsial infections) (Canadian Pediatric Society, 1994).

©1997 Ontario's Anti-infective Guidelines: TMP/SMX=Trimethoprim/Sulfamethoxazole

[‡] Common oral dosage ranges are provided unless otherwise stated. Consult the drug monogragh for details on age and condition specific dosing.
* Approximate costs were derived from the ODB formulary (# 35) or manufacturers' price lists and do not include professional fees or markups. **Page 36**

Modifying Circumstances	Probable Organism(s)	Antibiotic Choice(s)		Usual Dosage‡	Cost per day*

Bites - Human (For infected bites NOT prophylaxis)

Modifying Circumstances	Probable Organism(s)		Antibiotic Choice(s)	Usual Dosage‡	Cost per day*
HUMAN **INCLUDES CLOSED FIST INJURIES**	Viridans Strep Anaerobic streptococci Fusobacter	*FIRST LINE*	**Amoxicillin/Clavulanate**	250-500mg TID Children: 40mg/kg/day amoxicillin divided q8h	$2.62- $4.08 $0.15/kg
	S. aureus Bacteroides	*SECOND LINE*	**Erythromycin (for adults)** **Erythromycin estolate (for children)**	1g/day divided BID, TID or QID Children: 40mg/kg/day divided q6h	$0.21- $1.50 $0.03- $0.04/kg
			Clarithromycin	250mg BID Children: 15mg/kg/day divided q12h	$2.96 $0.09/kg
		THIRD LINE	**Clindamycin**	150-300mg QID Children: 20-30mg/kg/day divided q6h	$3.10- $6.21 $0.10- $0.15/kg

©1997 Ontario's Anti-infective Guidelines: TMP/SMX=Trimethoprim/Sulfamethoxazole

‡ Common oral dosage ranges are provided unless otherwise stated. Consult the drug monogragh for details on age and condition specific dosing.
* Approximate costs were derived from the ODB formulary (# 35) or manufacturers' price lists and do not include professional fees or markups.   *Page 37*

Modifying Circumstances	Probable Organism(s)		Antibiotic Choice(s)	Usual Dosage[‡]	Cost per day*

Lyme Disease [1,2,3,4]

Modifying Circumstances	Probable Organism(s)		Antibiotic Choice(s)	Usual Dosage[‡]	Cost per day*
ADULTS	Borrelia burgdorferi	FIRST LINE	(Amoxicillin +/-	500mg-1g TID	$0.62
			Probenecid) OR	500mg TID	$0.57
			Doxycycline [5]	100-200mg BID-TID	$3.40
		SECOND LINE	Cefuroxime -AX	500mg -1g BID	$11.48
		THIRD LINE	Ceftriaxone IV [6]	1-2 g q24h or 500mg - 1g q12h	$34.00- $67.00
CHILDREN	Borrelia burgdorferi	FIRST LINE	Amoxicillin PLUS	40mg/kg/day divided q8h	$0.03/kg
			Probenecid	40mg/kg/day divided q8h	$0.02/kg
		SECOND LINE	Cefuroxime-AX	30mg/kg/day divided q12h	$0.18/kg
		THIRD LINE	Ceftriaxone IV/IM [6]	50-100mg/kg/day divided q12-24h	$1.70- $3.40/kg

1) Adapted from Consensus Conference on Lyme Disease, 1991; Burrascano, 1996; Canadian Pediatric Society, 1992.

2) Reportable to Local Medical Officer of Health. Further information available from the Lyme Disease Association of Ontario at (519) 843-3646.

3) Lyme disease must be considered whenever neurologic disease occurs in association with significant constitutional or extraneural features. Neurologic involvement occurs in 10-40% of symptomatic infections and occur at all stages of infection. Patients with early local disease may experience mild headache, stiff neck, fatigue and myalgias. The dissemination stage is associated with certain neurologic syndromes that tend to improve spontaneously after several weeks to months without treatment. Cases have been documented in all regions of Ontario.

4) Duration of therapy is controversial. For early localized infection (single erythema migrans with no constitutional symptoms) treat six weeks. For early disseminated disease (multiple lesions, constitutional symptoms, lymphadenopathy, etc.) with mild symptoms present for less than one year: oral therapy until no active disease for 4 weeks (4-6 months typical). For late disseminated disease (symptoms greater than 1 year, more severely ill, immunocompromised) extended IV therapy (6-10 weeks) then oral or IM to same endpoint. Pulsed high-dose treatment has been successful in some patients who fail conventional therapy (cycle of treatment for 1 or 2 days, followed by no treatment for 6 days. Repeat 6 to 10 times). Note that infection may persist following treatment even when a patient becomes seronegative, and successfully treated patients may remain seropositive for years. Currently there is no test to confirm when all the Borrelia have been eradicated, so clinical follow-up assumes a major role in lyme disease (Coyle, 1993).

5) Tetracyclines increase skin/eye sensitivity to sunlight; advise patients to take proper precautions.

6) Ceftriaxone should be reserved for severe cases: CNS disease with CSF fluid abnormalities, high degree (2nd or 3rd) atrioventricular block, arthritis.

©1997 Ontario's Anti-infective Guidelines: TMP/SMX=Trimethoprim/Sulfamethoxazole

‡ Common oral dosage ranges are provided unless otherwise stated. Consult the drug monogragh for details on age and condition specific dosing.
* Approximate costs were derived from the ODB formulary (# 35) or manufacturers' price lists and do not include professional fees or markups.   Page 38

Modifying Circumstances	Probable Organism(s)	Antibiotic Choice(s)	Usual Dosage[‡]	Cost per day*

Herpes Simplex Virus - Mucocutaneous [1]
(Normal Host)

Modifying Circumstances	Probable Organism(s)	Antibiotic Choice(s)	Usual Dosage[‡]	Cost per day*
COLD SORES	Herpes Simplex type 1 or 2	No therapy recommended.		
LOCALIZED LESIONS		No treatment unless suspect dissemination, then use acyclovir.		
LOCALIZED BUT CHRONIC (PERI-ANAL)		Acyclovir oral may be useful.	200mg 5 times daily	$5.86
GINGIVAL STOMATITIS		No definitive recommendations available.		
ORAL LABIAL		No definitive recommendations available.		

(Immunocompromised Host) [2]

Modifying Circumstances	Probable Organism(s)	Antibiotic Choice(s)	Usual Dosage[‡]	Cost per day*
		No definitive recommendations available.		

1) Acyclovir topical is not an effective therapy.
2) No general guidelines for immunocompromised hosts. Individualize therapy and consult specialist as needed.

©1997 Ontario's Anti-infective Guidelines: TMP/SMX=Trimethoprim/Sulfamethoxazole

‡ Common oral dosage ranges are provided unless otherwise stated. Consult the drug monogragh for details on age and condition specific dosing.
* Approximate costs were derived from the ODB formulary (# 35) or manufacturers' price lists and do not include professional fees or markups.   *Page 39*

Modifying Circumstances	Probable Organism(s)		Antibiotic Choice(s)	Usual Dosage‡	Cost per day*

Herpes Simplex Virus - Adult, Genital Herpes [1]
(Normal Host)

Modifying Circumstances	Probable Organism(s)		Antibiotic Choice(s)	Usual Dosage‡	Cost per day*
1ST EPISODE [2]	Herpes Simplex type 1 or 2		**No treatment**		
SEVERE 1ST EPISODE		*FIRST LINE*	Acyclovir oral/IV	Oral: 200mg 5 times daily for 5-10 days or until healing complete. IV: 5mg/kg q8h	Oral: $5.86 1g vial: $138.98
			Valacyclovir	500mg BID for 5 days	$6.04
ACUTE RECURRENT < 6 EPISODES A YEAR			No treatment; acyclovir or valacyclovir is an option for severe cases. Initiate within 24 hours of onset.		
6 -12 EPISODES A YEAR WITH PRODROME		*FIRST LINE*	Consider episodic, early, patient initiated therapy with:	Initiate within 24 hrs of onset of rash	
			Acyclovir [3] OR	200mg 5 times daily for 5 days	$5.86
			Valacyclovir [3]	500mg BID for 5 days	$6.04
		SECOND LINE	Consider chronic suppressive therapy:		
			Acyclovir [4]	200-400mg BID to TID	$2.34- $6.78
			Valacyclovir	500mg daily	$3.02
> 12 EPISODES A YEAR		*FIRST LINE*	Consider chronic suppressive therapy: Acyclovir [4]	200-400mg BID to TID	$2.34- $6.78
			Valacyclovir	500mg daily	$3.02

(Immunocompromised Host)

Modifying Circumstances	Probable Organism(s)		Antibiotic Choice(s)	Usual Dosage‡	Cost per day*
		FIRST LINE	Acyclovir Consider episodic, early, patient initiated therapy.	200mg 5 times daily for 5 days or until healed. Chronic suppressive therapy may be preferable.	$5.86

1) Acyclovir and valacyclovir provide no protection to partners. Condoms advised.
2) Primary infections are frequently asymptomatic. The 'first' episode here includes symptomatic primary and nonprimary first episodes. A primary episode is the first clinically-evident episode in a seronegative patient; usual incubation for symptomatic primary infection is 2 to 21 days. Non-primary is first clinically-evident episode in a seropositive patient; short or long incubation (sometimes years), systemic symptoms unusual.
3) Acyclovir has shown variable clinical benefit, however valacylovir has shown significant benefit including shortening of the duration of lesions, pain and viral shedding (Spotswood et al., 1996).
4) Dosage and duration is unclear. Watch for breakthrough with lower dosage. If patient is symptom-free for 6-12 months reassess need for continuous therapy. Resistance is not currently an issue.

©1997 Ontario's Anti-infective Guidelines: TMP/SMX=Trimethoprim/Sulfamethoxazole

‡ Common oral dosage ranges are provided unless otherwise stated. Consult the drug monogragh for details on age and condition specific dosing.
* Approximate costs were derived from the ODB formulary (# 35) or manufacturers' price lists and do not include professional fees or markups. **Page 40**

Modifying Circumstances	Probable Organism(s)	Antibiotic Choice(s)	Usual Dosage‡	Cost per day*

Herpes Simplex Virus - Children, Genital Herpes [1,2]
(Normal Host)

Modifying Circumstances	Probable Organism(s)	Antibiotic Choice(s)	Usual Dosage‡	Cost per day*
1ST EPISODE PREPUBERTAL	Herpes Simplex type 1 or 2	Acyclovir is probably effective however there is no data to support its efficacy for this group.	Do not initiate if rash present longer than 72 hrs. 200mg QID for 5 to 7 days	$4.69
ACUTE RECURRENT		No data to support efficacy of acyclovir, although efficacy and safety are probably not different than for adults.	Must initiate within 24 hrs. of rash 200mg QID for 5 to 7 days	$4.69

(Immunocompromised Host)

Modifying Circumstances	Probable Organism(s)	Antibiotic Choice(s)	Usual Dosage‡	Cost per day*
		Acyclovir	Oral: 40-80mg/kg/day divided QID for 5 to 7 days IV: $500mg/m^2$ q8h for 5 days or until healing complete may be effective.	1g vial: $138.98
If acyclovir resistant		Foscarnet (investigational)	40-60mg/kg q8h	

(Chronic Suppressive Therapy)

Modifying Circumstances	Probable Organism(s)	Antibiotic Choice(s)	Usual Dosage‡	Cost per day*
		No data available		

1) There is no generally accepted consensus on the first line treatment.
2) Adapted from: Canadian STD Guidelines, 1995.

©1997 Ontario's Anti-infective Guidelines: TMP/SMX=Trimethoprim/Sulfamethoxazole

‡ Common oral dosage ranges are provided unless otherwise stated. Consult the drug monogragh for details on age and condition specific dosing.
* Approximate costs were derived from the ODB formulary (# 35) or manufacturers' price lists and do not include professional fees or markups.   Page 41

Modifying Circumstances	Probable Organism(s)	Antibiotic Choice(s)	Usual Dosage[‡]	Cost per day*

Herpes Simplex Virus - *Keratitis or Keratoconjunctivitis* [1,2]

Modifying Circumstances	Probable Organism(s)	Antibiotic Choice(s)	Usual Dosage[‡]	Cost per day*
ADULTS AND CHILDREN	Herpes Simplex type 1 or 2	**FIRST LINE** Idoxuridine 0.1% (HERPLEX)	Instill 1 or more drops every hour during waking hours. If severe lesions consider prn q2h during night. Cover adjacent areas. Wait a minimum of 24 hours after lesion has disappeared before discontinuing.	5ml: $13.18
		Trifluridine [3] (VIROPTIC 1%) ophthalmic solution	Instill 1 drop onto cornea q2h while awake. Maximum daily dose is 9 drops. Continue until lesion re-epithelialized then 1 drop q4h for 7 days.	7.5mL: $27.00

1) Consult an ophthalmologist.
2) Do not use any steroid containing preparation.
3) Administration of a full dosage regimen for periods exceeding 21 days should be avoided because of potential ocular toxicity.

©1997 Ontario's Anti-infective Guidelines: TMP/SMX=Trimethoprim/Sulfamethoxazole

‡ Common oral dosage ranges are provided unless otherwise stated. Consult the drug monogragh for details on age and condition specific dosing.
* Approximate costs were derived from the ODB formulary (# 35) or manufacturers' price lists and do not include professional fees or markups.   **Page 42**

Modifying Circumstances	Probable Organism(s)	Antibiotic Choice(s)	Usual Dosage‡	Cost per day*

Varicella (Herpes) Zoster Virus - Shingles
(Normal Host)

Modifying Circumstances	Probable Organism(s)		Antibiotic Choice(s)	Usual Dosage‡	Cost per day*
Mild to Moderate	Varicella Zoster		**No treatment recommended**		
Severe		*FIRST LINE*		Initiate within 72 hrs. of symptoms.	
			Valacyclovir [1]	1g TID for 7 days Children: not indicated	$18.12
			Famciclovir [1]	500mg TID for 7 days Children: not indicated	$20.40
		SECOND LINE	**Acyclovir** [1]	Initiate within 72 hrs. of symptoms. 800mg 5 times daily for 7-10 days. Children: 20mg/kg QID for 7-10 days	$22.16
		IV	**Acyclovir IV**	10mg/kg q8h or 30mg/kg/day Children: 250mg/m^2 q8h	1g vial: $138.98

(Immunocompromised Host)

Modifying Circumstances	Probable Organism(s)		Antibiotic Choice(s)	Usual Dosage‡	Cost per day*
		FIRST LINE	**Acyclovir IV** [2]	Should be initiated within 72 hrs. of symptoms. 10mg/kg q8h or 30mg/kg/day	1g vial: $138.98
				Children: IV: < 1yr: 10mg/kg q8h	1g vial: $138.98
				IV: ≥ 1yr: 500mg/m^2 q8h	
				PO (following IV): 80mg/kg/day divided QID	

1) Postherpetic neuralgia is by far the most common complication of herpes zoster and is one of the most intractable pain disorders. Incidence, severity and duration of episodes increase with increased age. Nearly one-half of patients over 60 years of age have this complication. Famciclovir 500mg for 7 days is an effective well tolerated therapy for shingles that has been shown to produce a statistically significant reduction in the duration of post-herpetic neuralgia compared with placebo (Tyring, 1995). Valacyclovir has been shown to produce statistically significant reduction in the duration of post herpetic neuralgia compared with acyclovir in patients over 50 years of age (Beutner, 1995). The treatment of shingles with acyclovir is of very little value overall and of **no** value if initiated more than 72 hours following onset of symptoms. There has been no difference reported between acyclovir and placebo in decreasing incidence or duration of postherpetic neuralgia (McKendrick, 1989).

2) In certain circumstances oral famciclovir/valacyclovir may be appropriate (e.g. step-down from IV therapy).

‡ Common oral dosage ranges are provided unless otherwise stated. Consult the drug monogragh for details on age and condition specific dosing.
* Approximate costs were derived from the ODB formulary (# 35) or manufacturers' price lists and do not include professional fees or markups.

Modifying Circumstances	Probable Organism(s)	Antibiotic Choice(s)		Usual Dosage‡	Cost per day*

Varicella (Herpes) Zoster Virus - Shingles cont..
(V1 Zoster or Zoster Ophthalmicus)

Modifying Circumstances	Probable Organism(s)		Antibiotic Choice(s)	Usual Dosage‡	Cost per day*
NON-OPHTHALMIC OR OPHTHALMIC		*ORAL*	Valacyclovir	1g TID x 7 days	$18.12
			or	Children: not indicated	
			Famciclovir	500mg TID x 7 days	$20.40
			and consult ophthalmologist	Children: not indicated	
		IV	Acyclovir IV and consult ophthalmologist [1]	10mg/kg q8h or 30mg/kg/day for a minimum of 5 days Children: IV: $\geq$ 1yr: 500mg/m^2 q8h PO (following IV): 80mg/kg/day divided QID	1g vial: $138.98

‡ Common oral dosage ranges are provided unless otherwise stated. Consult the drug monogragh for details on age and condition specific dosing.
* Approximate costs were derived from the ODB formulary (# 35) or manufacturers' price lists and do not include professional fees or markups.   **Page 44**

Modifying Circumstances	Probable Organism(s)	Antibiotic Choice(s)	Usual Dosage‡	Cost per day*

Chickenpox [1,2]
(Normal Host)

Modifying Circumstances	Probable Organism(s)	Antibiotic Choice(s)	Usual Dosage‡	Cost per day*
ADULTS [3]	Varicella Zoster	Acyclovir	If treatment is to have any benefit initiate within 24 hrs. of onset of rash 20mg/kg/dose (max. 800mg) 4 times daily for 5 days	$18.13
CHILDREN		**Acyclovir not recommended for routine treatment**		
DURING PREGNANCY [3]		**1. Do Serology (95% immune) following exposure to chickenpox** **2. Treatment: Acyclovir IV**	Acyclovir IV: $1500mg/m^2/day$ divided q8h for a minimum of five days	1g: $138.98
NEONATES [4]		**Prevention: VZIG** **Treatment: Acyclovir IV**	< 1 month of age: 30mg/kg/day divided q8h for 7 days	1g: $138.98

(Immunocompromised Host)

Modifying Circumstances	Probable Organism(s)	Antibiotic Choice(s)	Usual Dosage‡	Cost per day*
ADULTS		**Acyclovir IV**	10mg/kg q8h or 30mg/kg/day for 7 days	1g: $138.98
CHILDREN		**Acyclovir IV plus VZIG for prevention in children who have NOT had chickenpox.**	$1500mg/m^2/day$ divided q8h for 7 days	1g: $138.98

1) Reportable to the Local Medical Officer of Health.
2) Adapted from the Canadian Paediatric Society Statement: Chickenpox: Prevention and Treatment, 1994.
3) **These are not recommendations for prevention of chickenpox, only for treatment after it has been contracted.** Because healthy adults and pregnant women are at greater risk of severe illness and death from chickenpox, VZIG (Varicella Zoster Immune Globulin) prophylaxis **may** be considered in susceptible adults with household or other close contact with a case of chickenpox. It should be noted, however, that although a number of references recommend this treatment, there is no evidence to support this. VZIG in pregnant women may mask the development of clinical symptoms of chicken pox, however it will not offer protection of the fetus. Where possible blood should be obtained to determine VZ antibody status since negative histories from adults about prior chickenpox are not very reliable (70% of those with negative history are also immune). A positive history is very reliable in indicating immunity.
4) Infants born to mothers who developed chickenpox within 5 days before to 2 days after delivery should receive VZIG as soon as possible after delivery in order to reduce the risk of severe or fatal chickenpox. If VZIG fails and chickenpox develops, the infant should be hospitalized and treated with Acyclovir IV 30mg/kg/day, divided into 3 daily doses for 7 days. Premature infants (< 28 weeks) born to mothers who have **not** had chickenpox and who are exposed to chickenpox after birth and before 3 months of chronological age should receive prophylaxis with VZIG.

©1997 Ontario's Anti-infective Guidelines: TMP/SMX=Trimethoprim/Sulfamethoxazole

‡ Common oral dosage ranges are provided unless otherwise stated. Consult the drug monogragh for details on age and condition specific dosing.
* Approximate costs were derived from the ODB formulary (# 35) or manufacturers' price lists and do not include professional fees or markups. **Page 45**

Genitourinary Infections

Modifying Circumstances	Probable Organism(s)		Antibiotic Choice(s)	Usual Dosage‡	Cost per day*

*Acute Urinary Tract Infection - Adults:*Uncomplicated [1,2]

Modifying Circumstances	Probable Organism(s)		Antibiotic Choice(s)	Usual Dosage‡	Cost per day*
ACUTE CYSTITIS	E. coli S. saprophyticus	**FIRST LINE**	TMP/SMX	2 tabs BID or 1 DS tab BID.	$0.33
FEMALES > 12 YEARS	Other Gram -ve bacilli		Trimethoprim	100mg BID or 200mg daily	$0.55
			Nitrofurantoin [3]	50-100mg QID	$0.07- $0.08
					Macrodantin: $1.30- $2.29
				OR Macrobid 100mg BID	Macrobid: $1.23
		SECOND LINE	Amoxicillin [4]	250-500mg TID	$ 0.31- $0.62
			Ofloxacin [5]	200mg BID	$4.14
			Norfloxacin [5]	400mg BID	$4.36
			Ciprofloxacin [5]	250-500mg BID	$4.44- $5.01
		THIRD LINE	Cephalexin	250mg QID	$0.69
			Amoxicillin/Clavulanate	250-500mg TID	$2.62- $4.08

1) Acute cystitis is characterized by a normal genitourinary tract; limited morbidity; consistent microbiological spectrum.

2) A **three day** course of treatment is usually adequate for all agents listed except amoxicillin. Older post-menopausal women generally do well on short course therapy, but could require seven day therapy. If this therapy is unsuccessful, obtain a culture and consider a more prolonged course of therapy or altering therapy.

3) Macro-crystals may be better tolerated than micro-crystalline nitrofurantoin. Efficacy of Macrobid 100mg BID = Macrodantin 50 mg QID. Nitrofurantoin should not be used in infants < 1 month of age.

4) Amoxicillin is not first choice since 20-30% of bacteria are resistant; seven days of therapy are required if amoxicillin is used.

5) Fluoroquinolones are useful if patient is allergic or intolerant to other therapies.

©1997 Ontario's Anti-infective Guidelines: TMP/SMX=Trimethoprim/Sulfamethoxazole

‡ Common oral dosage ranges are provided unless otherwise stated. Consult the drug monogragh for details on age and condition specific dosing.
* Approximate costs were derived from the ODB formulary (# 35) or manufacturers' price lists and do not include professional fees or markups.   **Page 48**

Modifying Circumstances	Probable Organism(s)		Antibiotic Choice(s)	Usual Dosage‡	Cost per day*

Recurrent Cystitis - Adults [1]

Modifying Circumstances	Probable Organism(s)		Antibiotic Choice(s)	Usual Dosage‡	Cost per day*
EARLY RECURRENCE <1 MONTH [2]	E. coli S. saprophyticus Other Gram -ve bacilli	FIRST LINE	TMP/SMX	2 tabs or 1 DS tab BID	$0.33
			Trimethoprim	100mg BID or 200mg daily	$0.55
			Nitrofurantoin [3]	50-100mg QID	$0.07- $0.08 Macrodantin: $1.30- $2.29
				OR Macrobid 100mg BID	Macrobid: $1.23
		SECOND LINE	Ofloxacin	200mg BID	$4.14
			Norfloxacin	400mg BID	$4.36
			Ciprofloxacin	500mg BID	$5.01
		THIRD LINE	Cephalexin	250mg QID	$0.69
FREQUENT RECURRENCE [4] 3 OR MORE EPISODES A YEAR [5]		FIRST LINE	TMP/SMX [6]	1 tab or 1/2 DS tab qhs or post-coital	$0.04
			Trimethoprim	100mg qhs or post-coital	$0.27
			Nitrofurantoin [3]	50mg qhs or post-coital	$0.02
				Macrocrystals 100mg qhs or post-coital	$0.57
		SECOND LINE	Cephalexin [7]	125-250mg qhs or post-coital	$0.09- $0.17
			Norfloxacin	200mg qhs	$1.09
			Ofloxacin	200mg qhs	$2.07
			Ciprofloxacin	250mg qhs	$2.22

1) Culture, re-assess for upper tract infection.
2) Re-treat for 10 to 14 days.
3) Macro-crystals may be better tolerated than micro-crystalline nitrofurantoin. Efficacy of Macrobid 100mg BID = Macrodantin 50 mg QID. Nitrofurantoin should not be used in infants < 1 month of age.
4) Alternate therapy for recurrent infection is short course self treatment if less than three infections per year.
5) Drug choice for recurrent infection should be based on cultures. Consider prophylaxis using continuous low dose or post-coital antibiotics if identified with intercourse. Patient should be re-assessed following six months of therapy. Women having frequent recurrences and who are not responding to therapy should be investigated. There is limited data available on the role of topical estrogens for post-menopausal women.
6) Long term low doses of TMP/SMX usually do not result in an increase of resistant flora.
7) Cephalexin is especially useful during pregnancy.

‡ Common oral dosage ranges are provided unless otherwise stated. Consult the drug monogragh for details on age and condition specific dosing.
* Approximate costs were derived from the ODB formulary (# 35) or manufacturers' price lists and do not include professional fees or markups.

Modifying Circumstances	Probable Organism(s)	Antibiotic Choice(s)		Usual Dosage‡	Cost per day*

Acute Cystitis in Pregnant Women [1,2,3]

Modifying Circumstances	Probable Organism(s)		Antibiotic Choice(s)	Usual Dosage‡	Cost per day*
	E. coli	FIRST LINE	Amoxicillin [4]	250-500mg TID	$ 0.31- $0.60
	Klebsiella				
	Proteus		Cephalexin	250mg QID	$0.69
	Enterococci				
			Nitrofurantoin [5,7]	50-100mg QID	$0.07- $0.08
					Macrodantin: $1.30- $2.29
				OR	
				Macrobid 100mg BID	Macrobid: $1.23
		SECOND LINE	TMP/SMX [6]	2 tabs BID or 1 DS tab BID	$0.33
			Trimethoprim [6]	100mg BID or 200mg daily	$0.55

1) Avoid using fluoroquinolones in pregnant women.
2) Do monthly follow-up cultures in pregnant women who are susceptible to recurrence.
3) A **three day** course of therapy is usually sufficient as long as a follow-up culture is obtained.
4) Treat with amoxicillin for 7 days.
5) Macro-crystals may be better tolerated than micro-crystalline nitrofurantoin. Efficacy of Macrobid 100mg BID = Macrodantin 50 mg QID. Nitrofurantoin should not be used in infants < 1 month of age.
6) **Avoid the use of TMP/SMX and trimethoprim during the last six weeks of pregnancy as these agents may displace bilirubin from albumin binding sites.**
7) **Nitrofurantoin is contraindicated in pregnant patients at term (36-42 weeks gestation), during labour and in neonates due to the possibility of hemolytic anemia.**

©1997 Ontario's Anti-infective Guidelines: TMP/SMX=Trimethoprim/Sulfamethoxazole

‡ Common oral dosage ranges are provided unless otherwise stated. Consult the drug monogragh for details on age and condition specific dosing.
* Approximate costs were derived from the ODB formulary (# 35) or manufacturers' price lists and do not include professional fees or markups.   **Page 50**

Modifying Circumstances	Probable Organism(s)		Antibiotic Choice(s)	Usual Dosage‡	Cost per day*

Acute Urinary Tract Infection - Children [1,2,3]

Modifying Circumstances	Probable Organism(s)		Antibiotic Choice(s)	Usual Dosage‡	Cost per day*
	E. coli Enterobacter Proteus Enterococcus	FIRST LINE	TMP/SMX	8-12mg/kg/day trimethoprim divided q12h	$0.02- $0.03/kg
			Nitrofurantoin [4]	5-7mg/kg/day divided q6h	$0.03- $0.04/kg Macrodantin: $0.04-0.06/kg
		SECOND LINE	Amoxicillin	40mg/kg/day divided q8h	$0.03/kg
			Cephalexin	25-50mg/kg/day divided q6h	$0.04- $0.07/kg
			Trimethoprim [5]	Not approved for children < 12 years 4mg/kg/day divided q12h	$0.01/kg
		THIRD LINE	Amoxicillin/Clavulanate	40mg/kg/day amoxicillin divided q8h	$0.15/kg
			Cefixime	8mg/kg/day divided q12-24h	$0.13/kg

1) Do not use fluoroquinolones in children.

2) Use seven to fourteen day course of therapy; short course therapy has not been shown to be effective in children under five years of age due to high incidence of reflux. Note that it is difficult to differentiate between upper and lower UTI in children.

3) **Reflux:** Children require investigation to detect abnormalities and may require long term antibiotic prophylaxis with nitrofurantoin or TMP/SMX until six months after refluxing stops. Counselling may be required for parents regarding the necessity of long-term therapy.

4) Nitrofurantoin is not active against *Ps. aeruginosa* or certain strains of *Klebsiella* and *Proteus*. Macro-crystals may be better tolerated than micro-crystalline nitrofurantoin. Nitrofurantoin should not be used in infants < 1 month of age.

5) Trimethoprim is not available in liquid form.

©1997 Ontario's Anti-infective Guidelines: TMP/SMX=Trimethoprim/Sulfamethoxazole

‡ Common oral dosage ranges are provided unless otherwise stated. Consult the drug monogragh for details on age and condition specific dosing.
* Approximate costs were derived from the ODB formulary (# 35) or manufacturers' price lists and do not include professional fees or markups. **Page 51**

Modifying Circumstances	Probable Organism(s)		Antibiotic Choice(s)	Usual Dosage‡	Cost per day*

Complicated Urinary Tract Infection - Adult [1]

Modifying Circumstances	Probable Organism(s)		Antibiotic Choice(s)	Usual Dosage‡	Cost per day*
ORAL THERAPY	Enterococci E. Coli Klebsiella Proteus Ps. aeruginosa Other Gram-ve bacilli	FIRST LINE	TMP/SMX	2 tabs BID or 1 DS tab BID	$0.33
			Trimethoprim	100mg BID or 200mg daily	$0.55
			Nitrofurantoin [2]	50-100mg QID	$0.07- $0.08
					Macrodantin: $1.30- $2.29
				OR	
				Macrobid 100mg BID	Macrobid: $1.23
		SECOND LINE	Amoxicillin/Clavulanate	250-500mg TID	$2.62- $4.08
			Ofloxacin [3]	200mg BID	$4.14
			Norfloxacin [3]	400mg BID	$4.36
			Ciprofloxacin [3]	500mg BID	$5.01
PARENTERAL THERAPY		FIRST LINE	Ampicillin IV PLUS ANY ONE of:	500mg q6h	$7.60
			Gentamicin IV [4]	4 to 6 mg/kg q24h	80mg: $4.17
			Tobramycin IV [4]	4 to 6 mg/kg q24h	80mg: $6.89
			Amikacin IV [4]	15-20mg/kg q24h	500mg: $29.25
		SECOND LINE	Cefotaxime IV	1g q12h	$18.40
			Ticarcillin/Clavulanate	3.1g q4-6h	$38.44 - $57.66
			Ceftriaxone IV/IM	1-2g q24h	$34.00 - $67.00
			Piperacillin/ Tazobactam	3g/0.375g q6h	$75.60
		THIRD LINE	Ceftazidime IV [5]	1-2g q8-12h	$37.70- $111.30
			Imipenem IV	500mg q6h	$98.68

1) Complicated UTI includes obstruction, chronic catheter, spinal cord injury, etc. It is characterized by multiple abnormalities, broad clinical spectrum, usually mixed bacteriology and generally more resistance. Clinical presentation is an important consideration. Culture and investigate any underlying causes. Treat for 10 to 14 days. Patients with catheters should not be treated unless there is evidence of systemic disease.
2) Nitrofurantoin is not active against *Ps. aeruginosa* or certain strains of *Klebsiella* and *Proteus* species. Macro-crystals may be better tolerated than micro-crystalline nitrofurantoin. Efficacy of Macrobid 100mg BID = Macrodantin 50 mg QID. Nitrofurantoin should not be used in infants < 1 month of age.
3) Avoid first line use of fluoroquinolones, reserve for when there is a high probability of resistant organisms.
4) Gentamicin, tobramycin and amikacin may be given q24h rather than the conventional dosing of q8h for short term use where there is normal creatinine clearance. If duration of therapy extends beyond 2 or 3 days check creatinine clearance. With continued use beyond 5 days increased surveillance is recommended due to the potential for nephrotoxicity and ototoxicity, especially in elderly patients (otoxicity manifests either with dizziness/imbalance or hearing loss initially, depending on the aminoglycoside). For more information see page 90 or consider consulting a specialist.
5) Ceftazidime should only be used if Ps. aeruginosa is a consideration.

©1997 Ontario's Anti-infective Guidelines: TMP/SMX=Trimethoprim/Sulfamethoxazole

‡ Common oral dosage ranges are provided unless otherwise stated. Consult the drug monogragh for details on age and condition specific dosing.
* Approximate costs were derived from the ODB formulary (# 35) or manufacturers' price lists and do not include professional fees or markups.   Page 52

Modifying Circumstances	Probable Organism(s)	Antibiotic Choice(s)	Usual Dosage‡	Cost per day*

Asymptomatic Bacteriuria [1]

Modifying Circumstances	Probable Organism(s)		Antibiotic Choice(s)	Usual Dosage‡	Cost per day*
TREAT ONLY DURING PREGNANCY	Gram -ve bacilli Strep. Group B	FIRST LINE	Amoxicillin	250mg TID	$ 0.31
			Nitrofurantoin [2,3]	50-100mg QID	$0.07- $0.08 Macrodantin: $1.30- $2.29
			OR Macrobid 100mg BID		Macrobid: $1.23
		SECOND LINE	TMP/SMX [4]	2 tabs BID or 1 DS tab BID.	$0.33
			Cephalexin	250mg QID	$0.69

1) There are **no** indications for screening or therapy for asymptomatic UTI other than pregnancy and pre-operative G.U. procedures. **Pregnancy:** Screen once at 12-16 weeks. Treat with three day course, follow-up culture and repeat culture monthly; retreat if necessary. **Do not use** fluoroquinolones or tetracycline in pregnancy.
2) Macro-crystals may be better tolerated than micro-crystalline nitrofurantoin. Efficacy of Macrobid 100mg BID = Macrodantin 50 mg QID. Nitrofurantoin should not be used in infants < 1 month of age.
3) **Nitrofurantoin is contraindicated in pregnant patients at term (36-42 weeks gestation), during labour and in neonates due to the possibility of hemolytic anemia.**
4) **Avoid the use of TMP/SMX during the last six weeks of pregnancy as these agents may displace bilirubin from albumin binding sites.**

Chronic Urinary Tract Infection - Adult [1,2]

Modifying Circumstances	Probable Organism(s)	Antibiotic Choice(s)	Usual Dosage‡	Cost per day*
ELDERLY, NURSING HOME, NON-CATHETER		**Antibiotics not indicated**		

1) Antibiotics should only be used for symptomatic urinary tract infection. Asymptomatic bacteruria should not be treated. Chronic UTI may be symptomatic or asymptomatic. To make a diagnosis of UTI there must be > 10^8 cfu/ml and for asymptomatic bacteruria this must be on two consecutive specimens. Increased incontinence may be a manifestation of symptomatic urinary infection, but the presence or absence of incontinence has no bearing on asymptomatic bacteruria.
2) Elderly with chronic UTI may benefit from the use of a urinary antiseptic (e.g. methenamine hippurate 1g BID)

©1997 Ontario's Anti-infective Guidelines: TMP/SMX=Trimethoprim/Sulfamethoxazole

‡ Common oral dosage ranges are provided unless otherwise stated. Consult the drug monogragh for details on age and condition specific dosing.
* Approximate costs were derived from the ODB formulary (# 35) or manufacturers' price lists and do not include professional fees or markups.   **Page 53**

Modifying Circumstances	Probable Organism(s)		Antibiotic Choice(s)	Usual Dosage[‡]	Cost per day*

Pyelonephritis [1]

Modifying Circumstances	Probable Organism(s)		Antibiotic Choice(s)	Usual Dosage	Cost per day
NON-OBSTRUCTIVE	E. coli K. pneumoniae	*FIRST LINE*	TMP/SMX	2 tabs BID or 1 DS tab BID	$0.33
	Enterobacter		Trimethoprim	100mg BID or 200mg daily	$0.55
	P. mirabilis		Ofloxacin	200mg BID	$4.14
	Enterococcus faecalis		Norfloxacin	400mg BID	$4.36
	S. saprophyticus		Ciprofloxacin	250-500mg BID	$4.44- $5.01
			(Gentamicin IV [2]	4 to 6 mg/kg q24h	80mg vial: $4.17
			+/-		
			Ampicillin IV [3])	1-2g q4h	$10.60- $31.80
		SECOND LINE	Amoxicillin/Clavulanate	250-500mg TID	$2.62- $4.08
			TMP/SMX IV	4-5mg/kg q6-12h	5mL vial: $5.75
		THIRD LINE	Ciprofloxacin IV	400mg q12h	$66.00
COMPLICATED			**Refer to Complicated Urinary Tract Infections**		

1) Culture required. **Treat with fourteen day course of therapy**. Intravenous therapy may be necessary depending on clinical presentation (i.e. nausea and vomiting). Note that there are many other oral and IV agents that may be indicated.

2) Gentamicin may be given q24h rather than the conventional dosing of q8h for short term use where there is normal creatinine clearance. If duration of therapy extends beyond 2 or 3 days check creatinine clearance. With continued use beyond 5 days increased surveillance is recommended due to the potential for nephrotoxicity and ototoxicity, especially in elderly patients (otoxicity manifests either with dizziness/imbalance or hearing loss initially, depending on the aminoglycoside). For more information see page 90 or consider consulting a specialist.

3) If initiating treatment with parenteral therapy switch to oral therapy after three or four days. Diabetics and pregnant women are more susceptible to Strep. Group B and require ampicillin to be added empirically.

©1997 Ontario's Anti-infective Guidelines: TMP/SMX=Trimethoprim/Sulfamethoxazole

‡ Common oral dosage ranges are provided unless otherwise stated. Consult the drug monogragh for details on age and condition specific dosing.
* Approximate costs were derived from the ODB formulary (# 35) or manufacturers' price lists and do not include professional fees or markups. *Page 54*

Modifying Circumstances	Probable Organism(s)		Antibiotic Choice(s)	Usual Dosage‡	Cost per day*

Prostatitis - Acute [1,2]

Modifying Circumstances	Probable Organism(s)		Antibiotic Choice(s)	Usual Dosage‡	Cost per day*
MOST LIKELY BACTERIAL	E. coli S. aureus	*FIRST LINE*	**TMP/SMX**	2 tabs BID or 1 DS tab BID	$0.33
MILD TO MODERATE	Other Gram -ve bacilli		**Trimethoprim**	100mg BID or 200mg daily	$0.55
	Enterococcus faecalis		**Norfloxacin**	400mg BID	$4.36
			Ofloxacin	300mg BID	$4.86
			Ciprofloxacin	500mg BID	$5.01
		SECOND LINE	**Erythromycin**	1g/day divided BID, TID or QID	$0.21- $1.50
			Clarithromycin	500mg BID	$5.92
SEVERE		*FIRST LINE*	**Ampicillin IV**	500mg q6h	1g vial: $2.65
			PLUS ANY ONE of the following: **Gentamicin IV** [3] OR	 4 to 6 mg/kg q24h	 80mg vial: $4.17
			Tobramycin IV [3] OR	4 to 6mg/kg q24h	80mg vial: $6.89
			Amikacin IV [3]	15-20mg/kg q24h	500mg vial: $29.25

1) **Treat from four to six weeks**, if no evidence of improvement after two weeks, then re-assess. In older men with relapsing UTI the prostate is often the source. Acute prostatitis, although very rarely, can occur in prepubertal boys.

2) Patient may not be able to void in which case hospitalization and catheterization maybe be necessary.

3) Gentamicin, tobramycin and amikacin may be given q24h rather than the conventional dosing of q8h for short term use where there is normal creatinine clearance. If duration of therapy extends beyond 2 or 3 days check creatinine clearance. With continued use beyond 5 days increased surveillance is recommended due to the potential for nephrotoxicity and ototoxicity, especially in elderly patients (ototoxicity manifests either with dizziness/imbalance or hearing loss initially, depending on the aminoglycoside). For more information see page 90 or consider consulting a specialist.

©1997 Ontario's Anti-infective Guidelines: TMP/SMX=Trimethoprim/Sulfamethoxazole

‡ Common oral dosage ranges are provided unless otherwise stated. Consult the drug monogragh for details on age and condition specific dosing.
* Approximate costs were derived from the ODB formulary (# 35) or manufacturers' price lists and do not include professional fees or markups.   *Page 55*

Modifying Circumstances	Probable Organism(s)		Antibiotic Choice(s)	Usual Dosage‡	Cost per day*

Prostatitis - Chronic [1]

Modifying Circumstances	Probable Organism(s)		Antibiotic Choice(s)	Usual Dosage‡	Cost per day*
	E. coli Other Gram -ve bacilli	*FIRST LINE*	TMP/SMX	2 tabs BID or 1 DS tab BID.	$0.33
	Enterococcus faecalis		Trimethoprim	100mg BID or 200mg daily	$0.55
	Ps. aeruginosa	*SECOND LINE*	Erythromycin	1g/day divided BID, TID or QID	$0.21- $1.50
			Doxycycline	100mg BID	$3.40
			Norfloxacin	400mg BID	$4.36
			Ofloxacin	300mg BID	$4.86
			Ciprofloxacin	500mg BID	$5.01

1) This is a very difficult diagnostic category. Chronic bacterial prostatitis is characterized by recurrent episodes of bacteruria due to the same organism; chronic non-bacterial prostatitis is of unknown etiology and does not respond to antibiotics. When treating chronic prostatitis, cultures may be negative but clinical presentation significant; best to treat with syndrome approach. If there is no response in four to six weeks, chronic patients should be referred to a urologist. Chronic cases are less likely to be true bacterial prostatitis. Counsel patients to avoid excessive alcohol, spicy foods, caffeine, and chocolate. Increased sexual activity may reduce pain.

‡ Common oral dosage ranges are provided unless otherwise stated. Consult the drug monogragh for details on age and condition specific dosing.
* Approximate costs were derived from the ODB formulary (# 35) or manufacturers' price lists and do not include professional fees or markups.

Modifying Circumstances	Probable Organism(s)		Antibiotic Choice(s)	Usual Dosage‡	Cost per day*

Epididymitis - *Non-sexually Transmitted* [1,2]

Modifying Circumstances	Probable Organism(s)		Antibiotic Choice(s)	Usual Dosage‡	Cost per day*
USUALLY MEN > 35 YEARS	E. coli Other Gram -ve bacilli	*FIRST LINE*	TMP/SMX	2 tabs BID or 1 DS tab BID.	$0.33
		SECOND LINE	Cephalexin	250mg QID	$0.69
			Ofloxacin	200mg BID	$4.14
			Norfloxacin	400mg BID	$4.36
			Ciprofloxacin	250-500mg BID	$4.44- $5.01
		THIRD LINE	Gentamicin IV/IM PLUS	4 to 6 mg/kg q8h	80mg vial: $4.17
			Ampicillin IV	1-2g q4-6h	$10.60- $31.80

1) An anti-inflammatory medication may be indicated.
2) Presents as inflammation of the epididymis manifested by acute onset of unilateral testicular pain and swelling, often with tenderness of the vas deferens with erythema and edema of the overlying skin. This does not usually occur in prepubertal boys. It is very important to rule out torsion of the testes in both prepubertal and adolescent males if this diagnosis is being considered since this is a surgical emergency. (Canadian STD Guidelines, 1995)

©1997 Ontario's Anti-infective Guidelines: TMP/SMX=Trimethoprim/Sulfamethoxazole

‡ Common oral dosage ranges are provided unless otherwise stated. Consult the drug monogragh for details on age and condition specific dosing.
* Approximate costs were derived from the ODB formulary (# 35) or manufacturers' price lists and do not include professional fees or markups.   *Page 57*

Modifying Circumstances	Probable Organism(s)		Antibiotic Choice(s)	Usual Dosage[‡]	Cost per day*

Epididymitis - Sexually Transmitted [1,2,3]

Modifying Circumstances	Probable Organism(s)		Antibiotic Choice(s)	Usual Dosage[‡]	Cost per day*
USUALLY IN SEXUALLY ACTIVE MEN ≤ 35 YEARS	N. gonorrhoeae C. trachomatis	*FIRST LINE*	Ofloxacin [4] OR	400mg single dose	$2.43
			Ciprofloxacin [4] OR	500mg single dose	$2.51
			Cefixime OR	400mg single dose	$3.09
			Ceftriaxone IM	250mg single dose	$10.75
			ANY ONE of the above PLUS one of:		
			Tetracycline OR	500mg QID for 10 days	10 days: $1.60
			Doxycycline	100mg BID for 10 days	10 days: $34.00
	Treatment if due to C. trachomatis alone [5]	*FIRST LINE*	Tetracycline	500mg QID for 10 days	10 days: $1.60
			Doxycycline	100mg BID for 10 days	10 days: $34.00
		SECOND LINE	Erythromycin	2g/day in divided doses for 7 days. If not tolerated then 1g/day in divided doses for 14 days	7 days: $2.94- $21.00
			Ofloxacin	300mg BID for 7 days	7 days: $34.05
			Sulfamethoxazole	1g BID for 10 days	10 days: $4.21
			Azithromycin	1g orally single dose	$19.72

1) Adapted from the Canadian STD Guidelines, 1995. Must be reported to Medical Officer of Health.
2) Treatment is for epididymitis due to N. gonorrhoeae and C. trachomatis or if results are not available and urethral discharge is detected. Note that when epididymitis is accompanied by urethritis, it is presumed to be a sexually acquired infection, however, the urethritis may be asymptomatic and, therefore, overlooked. If neither smear nor urine shows PMN's defer antimicrobial treatment and immediately re-evaluate for torsion of the testicle.
3) An anti-inflammatory medication may be indicated.
4) Ciprofloxacin and ofloxacin should not be used if there is a possibility that the infection was acquired in Southeast Asia. If either of these agents is used in such a case a test-of-cure is recommended.
5) Smear of urethral secretions shows a mean of ≥ 4 polymorphonuclear leucocytes (PMNs)/field (x1000) but **no** gram-negative intracellular diplococci.

©1997 Ontario's Anti-infective Guidelines: TMP/SMX=Trimethoprim/Sulfamethoxazole

‡ Common oral dosage ranges are provided unless otherwise stated. Consult the drug monogragh for details on age and condition specific dosing.
* Approximate costs were derived from the ODB formulary (# 35) or manufacturers' price lists and do not include professional fees or markups.   *Page 58*

Modifying Circumstances	Probable Organism(s)		Antibiotic Choice(s)	Usual Dosage‡	Cost per day*

Pelvic Inflammatory Disease - Outpatient [1,2]

Modifying Circumstances	Probable Organism(s)		Antibiotic Choice(s)	Usual Dosage‡	Cost per day*
MILD TO MODERATE PRESENTATION	N. gonorrhoeae C. trachomatis	FIRST LINE	Ceftriaxone IM	250mg single dose	$10.75
			PLUS		
	M. hominis		Doxycycline	100mg BID for 14 days	14 days: $47.60
	Anaerobes	SECOND LINE	Doxycycline	100mg BID for 14 days	14 days: $47.60
	Coliforms		PLUS ANY ONE of the following:		
			Ofloxacin	400mg single dose	$2.43
			Ciprofloxacin	500mg single dose	$2.51
			Cefixime	400mg single dose	$3.09
IF GONOCOCCAL [3]		FIRST LINE	Doxycycline	100mg BID for 14 days	14 days: $47.60
			PLUS ANY ONE of:		
			Ofloxacin	400mg BID for 14 days	14 days: $68.04
			OR		
			Ciprofloxacin	500mg BID for 14 days	14 days: $70.16
			OR		
			Cefixime	400mg BID for 14 days	14 days: $86.52

1) Adapted from the Canadian STD Guidelines, 1995. Reportable to the Medical Officer of Health.

2) **Early treatment is essential**. All patients treated as outpatients should be re-evaluated 48-72 hours after the initial assessment and if their condition has not improved they should be admitted to hospital and a specialist consulted. Women who have had an episode of PID have a ten fold increased risk of subsequent PID, an 8-fold increased risk of ectopic pregnancy and a 10-fold increased risk of infertility.

Symptoms include: low abdominal pain of recent onset, metrorrhagia, intermenstrual or post coital vaginal bleeding, vaginal discharge that is not explained.

Signs: cervical motion tenderness, adnexal tenderness on bimanual examination (with or without a mass), cervicitis (purulent cervical exudate present in 30% of cases), fever (<40% of cases).

Pregnancy: Pregnant patients require hospitalization to evaluate other causes since PID is rare after the first trimester. Doxycycline should be replaced with erythromycin when treating pregnant patients.

Patients with IUD: IUD should be removed after therapy is initiated and patient is responding, unless the risk of pregnancy is high. Follow with contraceptive counselling.

3) Where gonococcal infection is diagnosed by Gram stain or culture or where there is an increased risk of gonococcal infection (street youth, previous STD, sexual contact with person with proven infection or compatible syndrome).

©1997 Ontario's Anti-infective Guidelines: TMP/SMX=Trimethoprim/Sulfamethoxazole

‡ Common oral dosage ranges are provided unless otherwise stated. Consult the drug monogragh for details on age and condition specific dosing.
* Approximate costs were derived from the ODB formulary (# 35) or manufacturers' price lists and do not include professional fees or markups.   **Page 59**

Modifying Circumstances	Probable Organism(s)	Antibiotic Choice(s)		Usual Dosage[‡]	Cost per day*
Urethritis - Gonococcal [1,2]					
ADOLESCENTS AND ADULTS > 9 YEARS	N. gonorrhoeae	FIRST LINE	Ofloxacin [3] OR	400mg single dose Not approved for children	$2.43
	C. trachomatis [2]		Ciprofloxacin [3] OR	500mg single dose Not approved for children < 18 yrs	$2.51
			Cefixime OR	400mg single dose	$3.09
			Ceftriaxone IM	250mg single dose	$10.75
			ANY ONE of the above PLUS one of: Tetracycline OR	500mg QID for 7 days	7 days: $1.12
			Doxycycline	100mg BID for 7 days	7 days: $23.80
		SECOND LINE	Spectinomycin IM PLUS ONE of Tetracycline OR	2g single dose 500mg QID for 7 days	$14.77 7 days: $1.12
			Doxycycline	100mg BID for 7 days	7 days: $23.80
CHILDREN ≤ 9 YEARS		FIRST LINE	Cefixime OR	16mg/kg single dose (max 400mg)	$0.27/kg
			Ceftriaxone IM PLUS	125mg single dose	$10.75
			Erythromycin estolate	40mg/kg/day divided q6-8h for 7 days	7 days: $0.28/kg
		SECOND LINE	Spectinomycin IM PLUS	40mg/kg single dose	$0.30/kg
			Erythromycin estolate	40mg/kg/day divided q6-8h Maximum: 500mg QID for 7 days	7 days: $0.28/kg

1) Adapted from the Canadian STD Guidelines, 1995. Must be reported to Medical Officer of Health.
2) Because C. trachomatis is so often accompanied by N. gonorrhea it is recommended to routinely treat both pathogens concomitantly. Where lab results are not available and there is urethral discharge treat for both; where no urethral discharge is detected defer antimicrobial treatment until results are available. Note that infections may be present without symptoms/signs or PMN response but, if present, requires treatment.
3) Quinolones (ciprofloxin and ofloxacin) should not be used if there is a possibility that the infection was acquired in Southeast Asia. If either of these agents is used in such a case a test-of-cure is recommended.

©1997 Ontario's Anti-infective Guidelines: TMP/SMX=Trimethoprim/Sulfamethoxazole

‡ Common oral dosage ranges are provided unless otherwise stated. Consult the drug monogragh for details on age and condition specific dosing.
* Approximate costs were derived from the ODB formulary (# 35) or manufacturers' price lists and do not include professional fees or markups.   **Page 60**

Modifying Circumstances	Probable Organism(s)	Antibiotic Choice(s)	Usual Dosage‡	Cost per day*

Urethritis - Nongonococcal [1,2]

Modifying Circumstances	Probable Organism(s)		Antibiotic Choice(s)	Usual Dosage‡	Cost per day*
ADOLESCENTS AND ADULTS > 9 YEARS		FIRST LINE	Tetracycline	500mg QID for 7 days	7 days: $1.12
			Doxycycline	100mg BID for 7 days	7 days: $23.80
		SECOND LINE	Erythromycin	2g/day divided QID for 7 days. If not tolerated then 1g/day divided QID for 14 days	7 days: $2.94- $21.00
			Ofloxacin	300mg BID for 7 days	7 days: $34.05
			Azithromycin	1g orally in a single dose	$19.72
			Sulfamethoxazole	1g BID for 10 days	10 days: $4.21
CHILDREN ≤ 9 YEARS		FIRST LINE	Erythromycin estolate	40mg/kg/day divided QID for 7 days Maximum 500mg QID	7 days: $0.28/kg
		SECOND LINE	Sulfamethoxazole	75mg/kg/day divided BID for 10 days Maximum 1g BID	10 days: $0.16/kg

1) Adapted from the Canadian STD Guidelines, 1995. Must be reported to Medical Officer of Health
2) In **pregnancy,** first line therapy is erythromycin (adult dosage as above). Erythromycin estolate is contraindicated. Second line therapy in the first two trimesters is sulfamethoxazole (adult dosage as above) and in the last trimester it is amoxicillin 500mg TID for 7 days.

©1997 Ontario's Anti-infective Guidelines: TMP/SMX=Trimethoprim/Sulfamethoxazole

‡ Common oral dosage ranges are provided unless otherwise stated. Consult the drug monogragh for details on age and condition specific dosing.
* Approximate costs were derived from the ODB formulary (# 35) or manufacturers' price lists and do not include professional fees or markups.   Page 61

Modifying Circumstances	Probable Organism(s)	Antibiotic Choice(s)		Usual Dosage‡	Cost per day*

Vaginitis [1,2,3] *(Trichomoniasis)*

Modifying Circumstances	Probable Organism(s)	Antibiotic Choice(s)		Usual Dosage‡	Cost per day*
TREAT ALL CASES AND THEIR SEXUAL PARTNERS REGARDLESS OF SYMPTOMS	T. vaginalis	*FIRST LINE*	Metronidazole [4]	2g orally single dose	Treatment: $0.22
		SECOND LINE	Clotrimazole ovule	100mg intravaginally daily for 6 days	Treatment: $9.06
			Clotrimazole 1% cream	one applicatorful intravaginally daily for 6 days	Treatment: $9.06

1) Adapted from the Canadian STD Guidelines, 1995.
2) Inflammation of the vulva, vagina or both, and/or excessive vaginal discharge not due to cervicitis. Vulvovaginitis can be either infectious or non-infectious (hypersensitivity, trauma, excessive physiologic secretions). Note that T. vaginalis and HSV are most often sexually transmitted. Rule out cervicitis.
3) Intravaginal products: bedtime administration is preferable.
4) Two recent papers have shown that metronidazole is not associated with teratogenic effects (Burtin et al., 1995; Piper et al., 1993) and can be used at any time during pregnancy. Some experts recommend interrupting breast feeding until 24 hours after completing therapy. Advise patient NOT to take any alcoholic beverages during metronidazole therapy and for 48 hours post-treatment to prevent disulfiram-like reaction.

Clinical Clues [1]

	Predisposing Factors	Symptoms	Signs
Candidiasis	• often absent • current or recent use of antibiotics • corticosteroids • diabetes mellitus • HIV infection • pregnancy	• itch • external dysuria • vaginal discharge • dyspareunia	• erythema and edema of vulva, vagina and/or introitus • white, clumpy adherent vaginal discharge
Trichomoniasis	• sexual activity	• vaginal discharge • itch • introital dyspareunia	• frothy, offwhite-yellow vaginal discharge
Bacterial vaginosis	• often absent • more common if sexually active	• vaginal discharge • fishy odour • may increase after intercourse	• grey to white thin vaginal discharge, often copious

1) *Source: Canadian STD Guidelines, 1995.*

©1997 Ontario's Anti-infective Guidelines: TMP/SMX=Trimethoprim/Sulfamethoxazole

‡ Common oral dosage ranges are provided unless otherwise stated. Consult the drug monogragh for details on age and condition specific dosing.
* Approximate costs were derived from the ODB formulary (# 35) or manufacturers' price lists and do not include professional fees or markups. **Page 62**

Modifying Circumstances	Probable Organism(s)	Antibiotic Choice(s)		Usual Dosage[‡]	Cost per day*

Bacterial Vaginosis [1,2,3]

Modifying Circumstances	Probable Organism(s)	Antibiotic Choice(s)		Usual Dosage[‡]	Cost per day*
ASYMPTOMATIC	Mixed anaerobic/ aerobic	**FIRST LINE**	Treatment is unnecessary unless pregnant, pre IUD insertion, pre-surgery, pre-induced abortion		
SYMPTOMATIC		**FIRST LINE**	Metronidazole [4]	500mg BID for 7 days	$0.11
				or	
No treatment needed for male sexual partner				2g single dose	$0.22
			Metronidazole 0.75% gel	one applicatorful intravaginally BID for 5 days	$17.43/30g
		SECOND LINE	Clindamycin	300mg BID for 7 days	$3.10
			Clindamycin 2% cream	one applicatorful intravaginally daily for 7 days	$23.78/40g

1) Adapted from the Canadian STD Guidelines, 1995 and the Medical Letter, 1995.

2) The characteristic feature of bacterial vaginosis (B.V.) is that it is a noninflammatory condition of the vaginal flora. B.V. is recognized as one cause of prematurity and the Canadian STD Guidelines supports the treatment of B.V. for all pregnant women. B.V. is linked with gynecological risks which include PID, cervicitis, post operation infection and other STDs.

3) Intravaginal products: bedtime administration is preferable.

4) Two recent papers have shown that metronidazole is not associated with teratogenic effects (Burtin et al., 1995; Piper et al., 1993) and can be used at any time during pregnancy. Some experts recommend interrupting breast feeding until 24 hours after completing therapy. Advise patient NOT to take any alcoholic beverages during metronidazole therapy and for 48 hours post-treatment to prevent disulfiram-like reaction.

©1997 Ontario's Anti-infective Guidelines: TMP/SMX=Trimethoprim/Sulfamethoxazole

[‡] Common oral dosage ranges are provided unless otherwise stated. Consult the drug monogragh for details on age and condition specific dosing.
* Approximate costs were derived from the ODB formulary (# 35) or manufacturers' price lists and do not include professional fees or markups.   *Page 63*

Modifying Circumstances	Probable Organism(s)	Antibiotic Choice(s)	Usual Dosage[‡]	Cost per day*

Vulvovaginal candidiasis (VVC) [1,2,3,4]

Modifying Circumstances	Probable Organism(s)		Antibiotic Choice(s)	Usual Dosage[‡]	Cost per day*
ASYMPTOMATIC	Candida sp. and other	FIRST LINE	Treatment is unnecessary		
SYMPTOMATIC		FIRST LINE	Clotrimazole	500mg tab intravaginally single dose	Treatment: $9.06
				OR	
				200mg tab intravaginally daily for 3 days	Treatment: $9.06
			Clotrimazole 1% cream	one applicatorful intravaginally daily for 6 days	Treatment: $9.06
			Miconazole	100mg ovule intravaginally daily for 7 days	Treatment: $9.78
				OR	
				400mg ovule intravaginally daily for 3 days	Treatment: $9.78
			Miconazole 2% cream	one applicatorful intravaginally daily for 7 days	Treatment: $9.78
			Tioconazole 6.5% ointment	one applicatorful intravaginally single application	Treatment: $10.74
			Fluconazole [5]	150mg cap single dose (ORAL)	Treatment: $15.80
			Terconazole 0.4% cream	one applicatorful intravaginally daily for 7 days	Treatment: $17.52
			Terconazole	80mg ovule intravaginally daily for 3 days	Treatment: $17.52

1) Adapted from the Canadian STD Guidelines, 1995.
2) Inflammation of the vulva, vagina or both, itch, external dysuria and/or excessive vaginal discharge not due to cervicitis. Vulvovaginitis can be either infectious (Candida sp. and other yeasts, trichomonas vaginalis (p.62), mixed anaerobic/aerobic bacteria (p.63), herpes simplex virus (HSV)) or non-infectious (hypersensitivity, trauma, excessive physiologic secretions). Note that T. vaginalis and HSV are most often sexually transmitted. Rule out cervicitis.
3) Intravaginal products: bedtime administration is preferable. Several of these preparations are available as over-the-counter products.
4) Recurrent VVC requires investigation for underlying causes and different therapeutic strategies. Specialist advice may be required. Male sexual partner should only be treated if *Candida* balanitis is present- use miconazole or clotrimazole cream applied BID for 7 days.
5) Contraindicated in pregnancy

©1997 Ontario's Anti-infective Guidelines: TMP/SMX=Trimethoprim/Sulfamethoxazole

‡ Common oral dosage ranges are provided unless otherwise stated. Consult the drug monogragh for details on age and condition specific dosing.
* Approximate costs were derived from the ODB formulary (# 35) or manufacturers' price lists and do not include professional fees or markups.   *Page 64*

Modifying Circumstances	Probable Organism(s)	Antibiotic Choice(s)	Usual Dosage[‡]	Cost per day[*]

Cervicitis [1,2]

Modifying Circumstances	Probable Organism(s)	Antibiotic Choice(s)	Usual Dosage[‡]	Cost per day[*]
	C. trachomatis **FIRST** N. gonorrhoeae **LINE**	Ofloxacin [3]	400mg single dose	$2.43
		OR		
		Ciprofloxacin [3]	500mg single dose	$2.50
		OR		
		Cefixime	400mg single dose	$3.09
		OR		
		Ceftriaxone IM	250mg single dose	$10.75
		ANY ONE of the above PLUS:		
		Tetracycline	500mg QID for 7 days	7 days : $1.12
		OR		
		Doxycycline	100mg BID for 7 days	7 days : $23.80

1) Adapted from the Canadian STD Guidelines, 1995. Must be reported to Medical Officer of Health.
2) The criteria for defining cervicitis, especially when signs are minimal, are not yet well standardized. Generally, an inflammation of the cervix with a mucopurulent or purulent cervical discharge and with an increased number of polymorphonuclear leucocytes (PMNs). If lab results are not available, treat for mucopurulent cervicitis due to N. gonorrhoeae and C. trachomatis. Evaluation of smear for PMNs is not valid during menstruation. Cervicitis does not occur in prepubertal girls; the counterpart is prepubertal vaginitis.
3) Quinolone (ciprofloxin and ofloxacin) should not be used if there is a possibility that the infection was acquired in Southeast Asia. If either of these agents is used in such a case a test-of-cure is recommended.

©1997 Ontario's Anti-infective Guidelines: TMP/SMX=Trimethoprim/Sulfamethoxazole

‡ Common oral dosage ranges are provided unless otherwise stated. Consult the drug monogragh for details on age and condition specific dosing.
* Approximate costs were derived from the ODB formulary (# 35) or manufacturers' price lists and do not include professional fees or markups.   *Page 65*

Central Nervous System Infections

Modifying Circumstances	Probable Organism(s)		Antibiotic Choice(s)	Usual Dosage[‡]	Cost per day*

Meningitis - Adult [1,2]

Modifying Circumstances	Probable Organism(s)		Antibiotic Choice(s)	Usual Dosage[‡]	Cost per day*
PREVIOUSLY NORMAL HOST	S. pneumoniae N. meningitidis H. influenzae	FIRST LINE	Ceftriaxone IV [3]	2g q12h for first 48 hours then q24h	2g: $67.00
			Cefotaxime IV [3]	2g q6-8h	$55.20- $73.60
			Penicillin G IV	2-4 million units q4-6h	$5.55- $16.66
		SECOND LINE	Ampicillin IV	2g q4-6h	$21.20- $31.80
		THIRD LINE	Chloramphenicol IV	50mg/kg/day divided q6h	1g: $3.73
			Ceftazidime IV	2g q6-8h	$111.30- $148.40
IMMUNOCOM - PROMISED (TRAUMA, MALIGNANCY, NEURO - SURGERY, OTHER)	S. pneumoniae N. meningitidis H. influenzae Enteric gm -ve S. aureus Listeria monocytogenes	FIRST LINE	(Cefotaxime IV OR	2g q6-8h	$55.20-$73.60
			Ceftriaxone IV)	2g q12h for first 48 hours then q24h	2g: $67.00
			+/- Ampicillin IV	2g q4-6h	$21.20- $31.80
		SECOND LINE	TMP/SMX IV	4-5mg/kg/day divided q6-12h	5mL vial: $5.75
	Ps. aeruginosa [4]	FIRST LINE	Ceftazidime IV [4] +/-	2g q6-8h	$111.15- $148.20
			(Tobramycin IV [5] OR	4 to 6mg/kg q24h	80mg vial: $6.89
			Amikacin IV [5])	15-20mg/kg q24h	500mg vial: $29.25

1) Reportable to Medical Officer of Health. Contact an infectious disease consultant regarding prophylaxis with rifampin for close contacts.

2) If penicillin resistant pneumococcus is a concern consider using vancomycin 1g q12h with a third generation cephalosporin (ceftriaxone or cefotaxime).

3) Given that meningitis is a medical emergency, it may be useful to give ceftriaxone or cefotaxime and modify antibiotic therapy according to culture results.

4) If Ps. aeruginosa is suspected, ceftazidime with or without aminoglycoside should be used.

5) Tobramycin and amikacin may be given q24h rather than the conventional dosing of q8h for short term use where there is normal creatinine clearance. If duration of therapy extends beyond 2 or 3 days check creatinine clearance. With continued use beyond 5 days increased surveillance is recommended due to the potential for nephrotoxicity and ototoxicity, especially in elderly patients (otoxicity manifests either with dizziness/imbalance or hearing loss initially, depending on the aminoglycoside). For more information see page 90 or consider consulting a specialist.

‡ Common oral dosage ranges are provided unless otherwise stated. Consult the drug monogragh for details on age and condition specific dosing.

* Approximate costs were derived from the ODB formulary (# 35) or manufacturers' price lists and do not include professional fees or markups.

Modifying Circumstances	Probable Organism(s)	Antibiotic Choice(s)		Usual Dosage[‡]	Cost per day*

Meningitis - Children [1,2,3]

Modifying Circumstances	Probable Organism(s)	Antibiotic Choice(s)		Usual Dosage[‡]	Cost per day*
INFANTS 1 - 3 MONTHS	S. pneumoniae	*FIRST LINE*	(Cefotaxime IV [4]	200mg/kg/day divided q6-8h	$1.84/kg
	N. meningitidis		OR		
	H. influenzae		Ceftriaxone IV [4])	80-100mg/kg/day divided q12-24h (maximum 4g/day)	$2.72- $3.40/kg
	Listeria monocytogenes				
	Coliforms		EITHER of the above PLUS:		
	Strep Group B [5]		Ampicillin IV	200-300mg/kg/day divided q6h	$0.05- $0.24/kg
CHILDREN AND YOUNG ADULT **3 MONTHS TO 18 YEARS**	S. pneumoniae N. meningitidis H. influenzae	*FIRST LINE*	Cefotaxime IV [4]	200mg/kg/day divided q6-8h (maximum 8g/day)	$1.84/kg
			Ceftriaxone IV [4]	80-100mg/kg/day divided q12-24h	$2.72- $3.40/kg
		SECOND LINE	Chloramphenicol IV +/-	75-100mg/kg/day divided q6h	$0.28-$0.37/kg
			Ampicillin IV	200-300mg/kg/day divided q6h (maximum 10g/day)	$0.03/kg

1) Reportable to Medical Officer of Health. Contact an infectious disease consultant regarding prophylaxis with rifampin for close contacts.

2) Initial therapy should be 3rd generation cephalosporin until pathogen is identified and antibiotic susceptibility determined because of prevalence of penicillin-resistant pneumococci and meningococci. If penicillin resistant pneumococcus is a concern consider using vancomycin with or without ampicillin. Switch to penicillin G IV or ampicillin IV if organism is found to be susceptible.

3) Note: Dexamethasone (0.6 mg/kg/day IV divided q6h x 4 days) as an adjunct to antibiotic therapy may decrease hearing deficits and other neurologic sequelae in Haemophilus meningitis and possibly other types. The first dose of dexamethasone is preferably given before the first dose of antibiotic (Nelson, 1993.)

4) Ceftriaxone safety is not yet established in neonates therefore only recommended from 1 month to 12 years of age. Cefotaxime is approved from day 0 of life: in neonates a dosage of 100mg/kg/day divided q12h from 0-1 week and 150mg/kg/day divided q8h from 1-4 weeks is recommended. If weight is over 50kg use adult dosage.

5) Strep. Group B requires ampicillin to be added.

©1997 Ontario's Anti-infective Guidelines: TMP/SMX=Trimethoprim/Sulfamethoxazole

‡ Common oral dosage ranges are provided unless otherwise stated. Consult the drug monogragh for details on age and condition specific dosing.
* Approximate costs were derived from the ODB formulary (# 35) or manufacturers' price lists and do not include professional fees or markups. **Page 69**

Gastrointestinal Infections

H. pylori Positive Peptic Ulcer Disease [1,2,3]

FOUR DRUG COMBINATION OPTIONS	Duration	Cost of One Week Treatment
1. Bismuth subsalicylate [4] 2 tabs or 30ml QID 2. Metronidazole [5] 500mg BID 3. Amoxicillin 1g BID or Tetracycline 500mg QID 4. Cimetidine 400mg BID or Ranitidine 150mg BID or Famotidine 40mg daily or Nizatidine 300mg daily	1 week Antibiotic treatment may be preceded by acid suppression for 1 week and/or followed by acid suppression for up to 4 to 8 weeks	$16.74-$31.02
1. Lansoprazole 30mg BID or Omeprazole 20mg BID 2. Amoxicillin 1g BID 3. Metronidazole [5] 500mg BID	1 week	$43.10-$45.90
1. Lansoprazole 30mg BID or Omeprazole 20mg BID 2. Amoxicillin 1g BID 3. Clarithromycin 500mg BID	1 week	$72.64-$75.44
1. Lansoprazole 30mg BID or Omeprazole 20mg BID 2. Metronidazole [5] 500mg BID 3. Clarithromycin 500mg BID	1 week	$81.34-$84.14

1) **Who to treat:** recommended for treatment of non-NSAID, non-malignant duodenal or gastric ulcer in presence of *Helicobacter pylori*. Patients with initial presentation or with recurrent gastric or duodenal ulcer disease, including those who are receiving maintenance therapy should be treated. Gastritis and nonulcer dyspepsia in presence of *H. pylori* should not be treated. Compared with intermittent acid suppression, *H. pylori* eradication is a more effective therapy for ulcer healing and significantly reduces recurrence rates several-fold (Blaser, 1996; O'Brien, 1996; NIH, 1994; Medical Letter, 1996).
Diagnosis: Non-invasive tests such as serology and urease breath tests are recommended where available. Invasive tests require endoscopy but are definitive. Follow-up is essential for complicated (bleeding, perforation, stricture) or refractory ulcers but is controversial after the medical management of uncomplicated ulcers in patients who remain asymptomatic. Follow-up testing should be done no earlier that one month after stopping agents capable of suppressing *H. pylori*. To minimize the risk of recurrences patients should be advised to stop NSAID use, stop smoking and minimize the use of alcohol.
2) Bacterial resistance has been reported to metronidazole and clarithromycin, but not to tetracycline or amoxicillin. For patients with an H.pylori-positive ulcer recurrence choose an alternative regimen that does not include the same agents. Note that treatment failure is often due to noncompliance.
3) All H2 antagonists have similar ulcer healing rates and side effect profiles. Note that a proton pump inhibitor plus 2 antibiotics decreases time with ulcer by 12 to 13 days compared to H2 antagonist triple therapy but at an extra cost ranging from $64 to $108 per patient per year (O'Brien et al., 1996)
4) Avoid bismuth subsalicylate (Pepto Bismol) and antacids if severe renal impairment present (creatinine clearance < 30ml/ min).
5) Advise patient NOT to take any alcoholic beverages during metronidazole therapy and for 48 hours post-treatment to prevent disulfiram - like reaction.

Modifying Circumstances	Drug Choice(s)	Usual Dosage‡	Cost per day*

Traveller's Diarrhea-Treatment and Prevention [1,2,3]

Modifying Circumstances	Drug Choice(s)	Usual Dosage‡	Cost per day*
Mild to moderate diarrhea (up to 5 movements per day)	Bismuth Subsalicylate (PEPTO-BISMOL, generics)	2 tabs or 30 mL repeat q30 min. as needed Maximum: 8 doses/day (prevention: 2 tabs or 30 mL QID with meals and in evening)	Over-the-counter agent
	Loperamide (IMODIUM, generics)	4 mg STAT, then 2 mg after each loose stool Maximum: 8 doses/day	Over-the-counter agent
	Diphenoxylate plus atropine (LOMOTIL)	5mg (2 tablets) TID - QID Maximum: 20mg (4 tablets) over 24 hours in divided doses Adjust dosage downward as soon as symptomatic control achieved.	$2.51 - $3.35
Severe (associated with fever and bloody diarrhea [4])	TMP/SMX	1 DS tab BID for 3 days (prevention: 1 DS tab daily)	$0.19
	Ciprofloxacin	500 mg BID for 1 to 3 days (prevention: 500mg daily)	$5.01
	Norfloxacin	400 mg BID for 1 to 3 days (prevention: 400 mg daily)	$4.36

1) Mild traveller's diarrhea will usually resolve in 24 hours with antimotility agents and fluids. Symptoms persisting more than 2 weeks after return home should be investigated thoroughly. Prophylaxis should only be used in patients at risk of the complications of diarrheal illness. Drugs taken for prevention should be started on the first day in the area of risk and continued for 1 or 2 days after return home, to a maximum of 3 weeks total.

2) Maintenance of fluid balance is vital. Clear fluid diet of carbonated beverages, fruit juices, hot tea or purified water and salted crackers. Moderate diarrhea may benefit from electrolyte-containing solutions. Severe diarrhea, particularly in young children, requires careful fluid replacement with a solution of 3.5 g sodium chloride, 2.5 g sodium bicarbonate, 1.5 g potassium chloride and 20 g glucose in 1 L of water or commercial preparations (Pedialyte, Gastrolyte).

3) May consider adding antibiotics where moderate symptoms are present. A number of studies suggest a role for antimotility agents plus antibiotics for moderately severe afebrile nondysenteric diarrhea, especially when the antibiotic is given in a high loading dose. Combining loperamide and TMP/SMX resulted in 75% of subjects recovering from diarrhea within 12 hours as compared with 34 hours for placebo (Wright, 1995).

4) Avoid antimotility agents in this situation since the agents have been shown to prolong invasive infection with Shigella, Salmonella and Campylobacter (Wright, 1995).

Prophylaxis

Recommended Routine Immunization Schedules in Ontario
(Public Health Branch, Ontario Ministry of Health, Feb. 1996)

Table 1

Infants Beginning Series in Early Infancy	
Age	**Vaccine**
2 months ♥	DPT Polio + Act-HIB ™
4 months	DPT Polio + Act-HIB ™
6 months	DPT Polio + Act-HIB ™
after 1st birthday ♠	MMR
18 months	DPT Polio + Act-HIB ™
4-6 years ♣	DPT Polio
14-16 years ♦	Td Polio

Table 2

Children 1- 6 Years of Age Not Immunized in Early Infancy	
Visit	**Vaccine**
Initial Visit ♥	DPT Polio + Act-HIB ™ , MMR
2 months after 1st visit	DPT Polio
2 months after 2nd visit	DPT Polio
12 months after 3rd visit	DPT Polio
4-6 years ♣	DPT Polio
14-16 years ♦	Td Polio

Table 3

Unimmunized Children Aged 7 Years And Over, and Adults Not Immunized in Childhood	
Visit	**Vaccine**
Initial visit	Td Polio ■, MMR ♠
2 months after 1st visit	Td Polio
6-12 months after 2nd visit	Td Polio
Every 10 years thereafter	Td
Adults ≥ 65 years or older, those with ● chronic heart or lung disease, and others at high risk	Influenza vaccine every autumn Pneumococcal vaccine once

Interruption of vaccine series does not require restarting the series, regardless of the length of time elapsed since the last dose.

Recommended Routine Immunization Schedules in Ontario cont..

Diphtheria, Pertussis, Tetanus and Polio

♣ The 4-6 year (5th) dose DPT Polio in Tables 1 and 2 is **not** necessary if the 4th dose was given after the 4th birthday.

♦ The polio vaccine booster dose at age 14-16 years is not required if the child has completed a primary series and received one or more doses of OPV in the past. OPV was used routinely in Ontario from January 1990 through March 1993.

■ Immunization of adults against poliomyelitis is **not** routinely recommended. Adults at high risk of poliovirus exposure, however, should have received a primary series. Thereafter, booster doses of polio vaccine are recommended only for travellers to areas where poliomyelitis is epidemic or endemic. This booster dose may be given if 10 or more years have elapsed since their last dose of polio vaccine. Table 3 outlines the primary series for unimmunized adults.

Haemophilus b (Hib) vaccine

Act-HIB^{TM} should be reconstituted with DPT Polio and administered i.m.. The routine primary series for infants is a dose at 2, 4 and 6 months. The same infant Hib vaccine should be used for the first three doses of the primary series. A booster dose is given at 18 months of age.

♥ For children beginning their infant Hib vaccine series at 3 months age or older, the recommended schedule is provided in the "Indications and Usage" section of the Act-HIB^{TM} product leaflet. Hib vaccine is not routinely recommended for children aged 5 years and over.

Measles, Mumps, Rubella

♠ MMR vaccine must be given after the 1st birthday. All school pupils must have documented receipt of 2 doses of measles vaccine. Children vaccinated prior to the 1st birthday are not considered appropriately vaccinated, and may be suspended from the school. Adults born after 1956 without evidence of immunity against these 3 diseases should receive MMR. All women of reproductive age without evidence of rubella immunity should receive MMR .

Pneumococcal Disease

● A single dose of pneumococcal vaccine is recommended for those over 65 years of age, people with chronic heart or lung disease and others at high risk. It may be given at the same as influenza vaccine.

Hepatitis B

Since 1994/95, this vaccine is routinely provided to Ontario school pupils in grade 7. It is also available for certain high risk groups.

For more information: Canadian Immunization Guide, 4th edition, 1993
Health Canada
Local public health department.
CMA Journal, September 1996

Modifying Circumstances		Antimalarial(s)	Usual Dosage[‡]	Useful in the following regions

Malaria Prophylaxis [1,2,3]

Modifying Circumstances		Antimalarial(s)	Usual Dosage[‡]	Useful in the following regions
CHLOROQUINE SENSITIVE		Chloroquine phosphate (ARALEN, generics)	500mg (300mg base) once per week **Children:** 8.3mg/kg (5mg/kg base) once per week, up to adult dose	Caribbean, Central America, N. Africa, parts of the Middle east
MEFLOQUINE SENSITIVE		Mefloquine[4] (LARIAM)	250mg base once per week **Children:** 5-15kg: 5mg/kg/week 15-19kg: 1/4 tablet per week 20-30kg: 1/2 tablet per week 31-45kg: 3/4 tablet per week	Africa, Asia, South America, SE Asia, Middle East
MEFLOQUINE RESISTANCE OR CONTRA - INDICATED	*FIRST LINE*	Doxycycline [3]	100mg daily **Children older than 8 years:** 2mg/kg/day (max. 100mg/day)	Thai borders with Laos, Cambodia, Mynamar
		Primaquine phosphate [3,5]	26.3mg (15mg base) daily **Children:** 0.5mg/kg (0.3mg base/kg) daily	South Pacific, SA Asia, Central America
	ALTERNATIVE	Chloroquine phosphate	500mg (300mg base) once per week **Children:** 8.3mg/kg (5mg/kg base) once per week, up to adult dose	
		PLUS Proguanil (PALUDRINE)	100mg daily or 200mg daily chloroquine resistant $\geq$ 2yr : 25mg ; 3-6yr : 50-75mg	
		PLUS STANDBY Pyrimethamine/ Sulfadoxine (FANSIDAR)	Three 500mg tablets as a single dose for self <u>treatment</u> when medical attention not available **Children:** 1-3 yrs: 1/2 tablet; 4-8 yrs: 1 tablet; 9-14 yrs: 2 tablets single dose	*(Note resistance to Fansidar : S. Africa, Thai border, Amazon, SE Asia)*

1) Adapted from the 1995 Canadian Recommendations for the Prevention and Treatment of Malaria and Keystone, 1996. When determining if prophylaxis is important consider: malaria endemicity, season, altitude, degree of rural travel, preventive measures for mosquito bites, age, pregnancy, allergies and concurrent medications/illnesses. All travellers to an endemic area require prophylaxis and protective measures such as use of DEET insect repellents. Information on malaria prevention can be obtained from the Centres for Disease Control at (404)332-4555.

2) Begin drugs 1 week before (except doxycycline, which is started 1 to 2 days before) and continue until 4 weeks after leaving the endemic area.   If fever develops within one year, and particularly within 2 months, of returning the patient should be considered to have malaria, regardless of prevention and it should be treated as a medical emergency. Malaria CANNOT be diagnosed without a blood film.

3) For pregnant women and young children use chloroquine first line. Proguanil is safe for use in pregnancy. Mefloquine may be used in the second half of pregnancy and in children over 5kg (5mg/kg/week base). Women of child-bearing years should be advised to use contraception while on mefloquine and for 3 months after the last dose. Doxycycline is contraindicated in pregnancy and in children < 8 years and Fansidar should not be used in the last month of pregnancy and in those with sulpha allergy.

4) Mefloquine is contraindicated for those with a previous history of psychosis, seizure disorder and/or during the first half of pregnancy. Avoid use in individuals with cardiac conductive disturbances.

5) G6PD level must be normal. Check G6PD level before initiating therapy.

Prevention of Infective Endocarditis [1,2]

DENTAL AND UPPER RESPIRATORY PROCEDURES ORAL[3]	*FIRST LINE*	**Amoxicillin**	3g one hour before the procedure and 1.5g six hours after initial dose
	SECOND LINE	**Clindamycin**	300mg one hour before the procedure and 150mg six hours after initial dose
		Erythromycin	1g two hours before the procedure and 500mg six hours after the initial dose
PARENTERAL[3]	*FIRST LINE*	**Ampicillin**	2g IM [4] or IV thirty minutes before the procedure and 1g IV/IM six hours after the initial dose
		Vancomycin	Infuse SLOWLY over one hour beginning one hour before the procedure. No repeat dose necessary due to long duration of action
		Clindamycin	300mg IV thirty minutes before the procedure and 150mg IV six hours after the initial dose
GASTRO INTESTINAL AND GENITO URINARY PROCEDURES	*FIRST LINE*	**Ampicillin AND**	3g one hour before the procedure
		Gentamicin	1.5mg/kg IM [4] or IV (max dose: 80mg) thirty minutes before the procedure
	SECOND LINE	**Vancomycin AND**	1g IV infused SLOWLY over one hour beginning one hour before the procedure
		Gentamicin	1.5mg/kg IM [4] or IV (max dose: 80mg) one hour before the procedure; gentamicin may be repeated once eight hours after the initial dose but vancomycin does not need to be repeated.

1) Adapted from the American Heart Association, 1990; Durack, 1995; RCDS, 1995.
2) Prophylaxis is recommended for the following:
Procedures: those procedures likely to result in gum bleeding (includes professional cleaning), intraligamentary injections, surgery or instrumentation of the respiratory, gastro-intestinal or genitourinary tracts expose patients with predisposing cardiac conditions to a risk of developing infective endocarditis.
Conditions: prosthetic heart valves, previous bacterial endocarditis (even in the absence of heart disease), surgically constructed systemic-pulmonary shunts, most congenital cardiac malformations, rheumatic or other acquired valvular dysfunction (even after valvular surgery), mitral valve prolapse with valvular regurgitation, hypertrophic cardiomyopathy and immunocompromised individuals.
If you are unsure of the need for prophylaxis please contact an Infectious disease specialist.
3) Oral regimens are more convenient and safer. Parenteral regimens are more likely to be effective; they are recommended especially for high risk patients (e.g. prosthetic heart valves, previous endocarditis, or those taking continuous oral penicillin for rheumatic fever prophylaxis). Parenteral therapy may be repeated once, 8 hours after the initial dose OR alternatively amoxicillin 1.5 g orally 6 hours after the initial dose may be given.
4) IM administration should be avoided in patients receiving anticoagulation therapy.

Pediatric Dosages

	Initial	Follow-up		Initial	Follow-up
Amoxicillin	50mg/kg	25mg/kg	Erythromycin Ethylsuccinate or Stearate	20mg/kg	10mg/kg
Ampicillin	50mg/kg	25mg/kg	Gentamicin	2mg/kg	1mg/kg
Clindamycin	10mg/kg	5mg/kg	Vancomycin	20mg/kg	10mg/kg

Tuberculosis [1]

NINE STEPS TO PERFORMING, INTERPRETING, AND ACTING UPON THE MANTOUX TEST

STEP 1: Assign the patient to one of the following groups:

Group A: Healthy adult, screening situation	**Group B**: Healthy child or adolescent, screening situation
Group C: Adult, TB suspected because of symptoms	**Group D**: Child or adolescent, TB suspected because of symptoms

STEP 2: Between 48 and 72 hours after the intradermal injection of 0.1 ml (5 TU) of tuberculin reagent, determine the diameter of induration at the injection site. Measure carefully, in mm, with a ruler. The diameter of redness is not important.

If there is no induration at all, STOP HERE. If there is induration, Go on to Step 3.

STEP 3: Determine whether the induration is large enough to be called positive using the chart below. Note that the impact of previous BCG vaccination on the Mantoux test is minimal. Disregard the fact that a person has received BCG when interpreting the Mantoux.

Group A: Healthy Adult, screening situation	Group B: Healthy Child or Adolescent, screening situation
Criteria for Positive Mantoux Test: **≥ 5 mm induration = Positive** if either recent close contact of TB or HIV infected	Criteria for Positive Mantoux Test: **≥ 5 mm induration = Positive** if either recent close contact of TB or HIV infected or severely immunosuppressed.
≥ 10 mm induration = Positive if from TB endemic area (Africa, Asia, Latin American, aboriginal community), lives in nursing home or prison, underlying medical condition (cancer, diabetes, corticosteroids) or elderly.	**≥ 10 mm induration = Positive** if age is less than 4 years, or from TB endemic area (Africa, Asia, Latin American, aboriginal community), or underlying medical condition (cancer, diabetes, corticosteroids)
≥ 15 mm induration = Positive if there are no known risk factors	**≥ 15 mm induration = Positive** if age ≥ 4 years and there are no known risk factors
If the Mantoux is defined as positive, Go To Step 5	**If the Mantoux is defined as positive, perform a chest X-ray.** **If the chest X-ray is normal, Go To Step 8: Isoniazid Prophylaxis** **If the chest X-ray is abnormal (compatible with TB) Go To Step 9: Active TB**

Group C: Adult, TB is suspected because of symptoms	Group D: Child or Adolescent, TB is suspected because of symptoms
Criteria for Positive Mantoux Test:	Criteria for Positive Mantoux Test:
≥ 5 mm induration = Positive if in recent close contact of TB case, HIV-infected, or chest X-ray shows evidence of TB that was never treated.	**≥ 5 mm induration = Positive** if in recent close contact of TB or HIV infected or severely immunosuppressed, or clinical picture/chest X-ray highly suggestive of TB
≥ 10 mm induration = Positive as for Group A above	**≥ 10 mm induration = Positive as Group B above**
≥ 15 mm induration = Positive as for Group A above	**≥ 15 mm induration = Positive as Group B above**
If the Mantoux is defined as Positive, Go To Step 9: Active TB	**If the Mantoux is defined as Positive Go To Step 9: Active TB**

Note: A negative Mantoux never rules out TB

STEP 4: If Step 3 shows that the induration is too small to be called positive, record the diameter in mm and STOP HERE. Future Mantoux tests will be compared to this one, so recording the mm of induration and your interpretation are important.

STEP 5: Healthy adult with Positive Mantoux: is it new or long-standing?
For adults in Group A, you must decide what to do with the healthy person with a positive Mantoux. Using the criteria listed here, decide whether the Mantoux converted to positive in the remote past or within the past two years. Further action depends on when the person became Mantoux Positive.

CONVERTED TO POSITIVE WITHIN PAST 2 YEARS:

Characteristics: NO TB symptoms and at least ONE of the following is true:
- the previous Mantoux had no induration when performed 1 or 2 years ago
- the diameter of the Mantoux is now 15 mm greater than it was when last performed (10 mm greater if the person is less than 35 years old or immunocompromised)
- no previous Mantoux was performed and the patient's known TB contact was in recent past (the Mantoux is being done now because of the TB contact)
  If the person probably converted within the past 2 years, Go To Step 6

STEP 5: continued

CONVERTED TO POSITIVE IN THE REMOTE PAST:

Characteristics: NO TB symptoms, over 20 years old AND one of the following is true:
- had a known positive Mantoux of similar size in the past
- or the Mantoux diameter is now less than 15 mm wider than a previously indurated Mantoux (less than 10 mm wider in person under 35 years or immunocompromised)
- or lived in a region high TB endemicity in the remote past
- or successfully treated for TB in the past
- or Mantoux not done previously and there are no risk factors for <u>recent</u> contact with TB
   If the person is now well and successfully treated for TB in the past, STOP HERE.
   If the person has no symptoms of TB, Go To Step 7

STEP 6: Silent TB Acquired within the Past 2 Years (ADULTS)

This step is for adults who are well (no cough, fever, night sweats or weight loss), but it is reasonably certain that the Mantoux became positive approximately within the past 2 years. You must verify whether or not the Chest X-Ray is normal before proceeding further:
   If the person has normal Chest X-ray, Go To Step 8: Isoniazid Prophylaxis
   If the Chest X-ray is abnormal (compatible with TB), Go To Step 9: Active TB

STEP 7: Silent TB Acquired in the Remote Past (ADULTS):

This step is for adults who are well (no cough, fever, night sweats or weight loss), and it is reasonably certain that the Mantoux became positive more than 2 years ago. You must verify whether or not the Chest X-Ray is normal before proceeding:
   If the Chest X-ray compatible with TB, Go To Step 9: Active TB
   If the Chest X-ray is normal, you must consider the age of the person before deciding whether or not prophylactic isoniazid (INH) is indicated:

   If the person is greater than age 35 years, <u>and</u> well, <u>and</u> has a normal chest X-ray, all experts agree that no more needs to be done. STOP HERE.
   If the person is age 20 to 35 years, and well, and has a normal chest X-ray, most authorities <u>do</u> recommend INH prophylaxis. Other experts are concerned that the risk of life-threatening INH-induced hepatitis is too high to warrant giving INH prophylaxis to anyone over 20 years unless it is reasonably certain that the Mantoux became positive within the past two years. (The risk of developing clinically significant active TB is highest only within the first two years after the Mantoux becomes positive.)
   If you decide to give INH prophylaxis to young adults, Go To Step 8: Isoniazid Prophylaxis

STEP 8: Isoniazid Prophylaxis

If the person is well <u>and</u> has a normal Chest X-Ray, a 6-9 month course of prophylactic isoniazid (INH) may be indicated (note: 12 months of therapy is recommended for children, where there is a chest X-ray abnormality and in immunocompromised patients. If the person is HIV positive minimum treatment time is 12 months depending on immune status, but prophylaxis may be life long). Concomitantly, give pyridoxine (vitamin B-6) to adults to prevent INH-induced peripheral neuropathy.

Isoniazid	**10mg/kg once daily (maximum 300mg)**
Pyridoxine (Vitamin B-6)	**25mg daily**

Before starting INH:

- Take a baseline serum bilirubin and ALT.
- If ALT or bilirubin are abnormal, seek a specialist's advice about TB prophylaxis: do not give INH to a person with pre-existing liver disease.
- Warn the person about the risk of INH hepatitis (2% of people over age 35 years; increases with age)
- Alcohol may potentiate the liver toxicity of INH so warn patients to consume little or no alcohol.
- Tell the person to stop INH immediately and seek medical help if anorexia, abdominal pain or jaundice occur. **Anorexia is an important first symptom of INH hepatitis**, an entity that can be life-threatening.
- To ensure compliance, patients should be seen monthly while on INH.
- There is no need to monitor serum bilirubin or ALT as long as the person remains well.
- If there has been contact with a known case of INH-resistant TB, refer the case to a specialist.
- Don't forget to prescribe the Vitamin B-6, 25 mg daily.

STEP 9: Management of Active TB:

Patients in this group may be clearly unwell (cough, fever, night sweats, or weight loss) or have only mild symptoms. They must be investigated to confirm active TB infection (chest X-rays and TB smears and cultures which are obtained from infected sites including sputum, gastric aspirate in children, urine, pleural fluid, CSF, bone or joint fluid). If you determine that the person probably has active TB, a multi-drug regimen of TB treatment should be given for 6 to 9 months, depending on the drugs chosen. Such treatment should be given under the guidance of a specialist.

Never start a person with suspected active TB on one drug alone, drug-resistant TB can emerge after only a short period of single-drug therapy.

---

1) Adapted from Pennie, 1995 and Marrie, 1995.

REPORTABLE DISEASES

The following specified Reportable Diseases are to be reported to the Local Medical Officer of Health:

Acquired Immunodeficiency Syndrome (AIDS) Amebiasis
* Anthrax
* Botulism
Brucellosis
Campylobacter enteritis
Chancroid
Chickenpox (Varicella)
Chlamydia trachomatis infections
* Cholera
Cytomegalovirus infection, congenital
* Diphtheria
Encephalitis, including:
i. Primary, viral
ii. Post-infectious
iii. Vaccine-related
iv. Subacute sclerosing panencephalitis
v. Unspecified
* Food poisoning, all causes
* Gastroenteritis, institutional outbreaks
Giardiasis, except asymptomatic cases
Gonorrhea
* Group A Streptococcal infections, invasive
Group B Streptococcal infections, neonatal
* Haemophilus influenzae b disease, invasive
* Hemorrhagic fevers, including:
i. Ebola virus disease
ii. Marburg virus disease
iii. Other viral causes
Hepatitis, viral
* i. Hepatitis A
ii. Hepatitis B
iii. Hepatitis C
iv. Hepatitis D (Delta hepatitis)
Herpes, neonatal
Influenza

* Lassa Fever
Legionellosis
Leprosy
Listeriosis
Lyme Disease
Malaria
* Measles
Meningitis, acute
* i. bacterial
ii. viral
iii. other
* Meningococcal disease, invasive
Mumps
Ophthalmia neonatorum
* Paratyphoid Fever
Pertussis (Whooping Cough)
* Plague
* Poliomyelitis, acute
Psittacosis/Ornithosis
Q Fever
* Rabies
Rubella
Rubella, congenital syndrome
Salmonellosis
* Shigellosis
Syphilis
Tetanus
Trichinosis
Tuberculosis
Tularemia
* Typhoid Fever
* Verotoxin-producing E. coli infection indicator conditions including Hemolytic Uremic Syndrome (HUS)
* Yellow Fever
Yersiniosis

Note: Diseases marked * (and influenza in institutions) should be reported immediately to the Medical Officer of Health by telephone. Other diseases are to be reported by the next working day.

For more information please call: Your Local Public Health Department

Ontario Ministry of Health June 1996

Pediatric Dosage Table

Generic Name	Route	Dose	Interval
Acyclovir	PO	15-80mg/kg/day depending on indication	q6h
Acyclovir	IV	25-50mg/kg/day	q8h
Amikacin	IV/IM	15-20mg/kg/day * q24h dosing is suitable for children beyond the neonatal period	q8h or q24h
Amoxicillin*	PO	40-100mg/kg/day	q8h
Amoxicillin/Clavulanate*	PO	40-60mg amoxicillin/kg/day	q8h
Ampicillin	PO IV	50mg/kg/day 100-200mg/kg/day (Meningitis: 200-300mg/kg/day)	q6h q6h
Cefaclor	PO	20-40mg/kg/day	q8-q12h
Cefadroxil	PO	30mg/kg/day	q12h
Cefazolin	IV/IM	50-100mg/kg/day	q8h
Cefixime	PO	8mg/kg/day	q12-24h
Cefotaxime	IV/IM	100-150mg/kg/day (Meningitis: 200mg/kg/day) Maximum dose: 10g daily	q6-8h
Cefprozil	PO	15-30mg/kg/day	q12h
Ceftazidime	IV/IM	100-150mg/kg/day (Meningitis: 225mg/kg/day)	q8h
Ceftriaxone	IV/IM	50-100mg/kg/day (Meningitis: 80-100mg/kg/day) Maximum dose: 4g daily	q12-24h
Cefuroxime	IV/IM	75mg/kg/day (Meningitis: 200-240mg/kg/day) Maximum dose: 9g daily	q8h
Cefuroxime axetil	PO	30-40 mg/kg/day Maximum dose: 1g daily	q12h
Cephalexin	PO	25-100mg/kg/day	q6h

* Higher doses of amoxicillin are indicated for oral "step down" therapy after I.V. dosing, and where partially resistant streptococcus pneumoniae is suspected.

Pediatric Dosage Table cont...

Generic Name	Route	Dose	Interval
Chloramphenicol	IV/PO	50-75mg/kg/day (Meningitis: 75-100mg/kg/day)	q6h
Ciprofloxacin	PO/IV	20-30mg/kg/day **Not approved for children.** **Special cases exist. Do not exceed** **dosage of 500mg BID.**	q12h
Clarithromycin	PO	15mg/kg/day	q12h
Clindamycin	PO IV/IM IV/IM	10-30mg/kg/day 15-25mg/kg/day -mild-moderate 25-40mg/kg/day - severe	q6-8h q6-8h
Cloxacillin	PO IV	50-100mg/kg/day 100-150mg/kg/day	q6h q6h
Doxycycline	PO	2-4mg/kg/day **Should not be used in children** **under 9 years of age.**	q12h on first day; then ½ dose q24h
Erythromycin base	PO	30-40mg/kg/day	q6-12h
Erythromycin estolate	PO	30-40mg/kg/day	q6-8h
Erythromycin ethylsuccinate/ Sulfisoxazole	PO	Base on erythromycin component: 40mg/kg/day	QID
Flucloxacillin	PO	25-50mg/kg/day	q6h
Fusidic Acid	Topical	Apply sparingly TID-QID. If covered with occlusive dressing daily or BID	TID-QID
Gentamicin	IV/IM	4-6mg/kg/day (Cystic fibrosis: 7-10mg/kg/day)	q8h or q24h
Imipenem	IV	60-100mg/kg/day (Maximum dose 2g/day)	q6h
Mupirocin	Topical	Apply to affected skin	TID
Nitrofurantoin	PO	5-7mg/kg/day	q6h
Nitrofurantoin macrocrystals	PO	5-7mg/kg/day	q6h

Pediatric Dosage Table cont...

Generic Name	Route	Dose	Interval
Norfloxacin	PO	Adults: 800mg/day **Not approved for children.** **Special cases exist; do not exceed** **maximum adult dose of** **800mg/day.**	q12h
Ofloxacin	PO	Adult: 400-800mg/day. **Not approved for children.** **Special cases exist; do not exceed** **maximum adult dose of** **800mg/day.**	q12h
Penicillin G	IV	100,000 - 250,000 units/kg/day	q6-8h
Penicillin V	PO	25-50mg/kg/day	q6-8h
Pivampicillin	PO	40-60 mg/kg/day (Maximum dose 500mg BID)	q12h
Probenecid	PO	25mg/kg initially, followed by 40mg/kg/day	q6h
Rifampin		Over 5 years: up to 20mg/kg/day (Maximum: 600mg daily) **Prophylaxis: meningococcal** >1 month: 10mg/kg q12h x 2 days <1 month: 5mg/kg q12h x 2 days **Prophylaxis: H. influenza Type B** >1month: 20mg/kg q24h x 4 days < 1month:10 mg/kg q24h x 4 days	
Spectinomycin	IM	40mg/kg (Maximum 2g) single dose for S.T.D.	
Sulfamethoxazole	PO	75mg/kg/day	q12h
Tetracycline	PO	25-50mg/kg/day **Should not be used in children** **under 9 years of age.**	q6h
Ticarcillin	IV	50-200mg/kg/day (Maximum dose 300mg/kg daily)	q4-8h
Ticarcillin/Clavulanate	IV	200-300mg/kg/day Ticarcillin	q4-6h
Tobramycin Sulfate	IV/IM	6-7.5mg/kg/day (Cystic fibrosis: 7-10mg/kg/day)	q8h or q24h
Trimethoprim/Sulfamethox azole (Co-trimoxazole)	PO	8-12mg/kg/day trimethoprim (20mg/kg/day trimethoprim for Pneumocystis)	q12h q6h
Vancomycin	IV	40mg/kg/day	q6-8h
Vidarabine	Topical	Approx. 1 cm of ointment	q3h

List of Abbreviations

Cefuroxime-AX	Cefuroxime axetil
ER/SX	Erythromycin ethylsuccinate/Sulfisoxazole
TMP/SMX	Trimethoprim/Sulfamethoxazole
DS	Double Strength
BID	Twice daily
TID	Three times daily
QID	Four times daily
qhs	At bedtime
PO	Oral
IM	Intramuscular
IV	Intravenously
ung	Ointment

Trade Name/Generic Name Listing

TRADE NAME	GENERIC NAME
BACTROBAN	Mupirocin
BIAXIN	Clarithromycin
CECLOR	Cefaclor
CEFTIN	Cefuroxime axetil
CEFZIL	Cefoprozil
CIPRO	Ciprofloxacin
CLAVULIN	Amoxicillin/Clavulanate
FAMVIR	Famciclovir
FLOXIN	Ofloxacin
FLUCLOX	Flucloxacillin
FUCIDIN	Fusidic Acid
NOROXIN	Norfloxacin
PEDIAZOLE	Erythromycin ethylsuccinate/Sulfisoxazole
PIPRACIL	Piperacillin
PONDOCILLIN	Pivampicillin
SUPRAX	Cefixime
TAZOCIN	Piperacillin/Tazobactam
VALTREX	Valacyclovir
ZITHROMAX	Azithromycin
ZOVIRAX	Acyclovir

Once Daily Aminoglycoside Dosing

All patients should receive once-daily aminoglycoside dosing except: pregnant women, neonates, patients with enterococcal endocarditis, ascites or osteomyelitis, patients receiving dialysis, for surgical prophylaxis or where febrile neutropenia is present.

Aminoglycosides can be given once daily without compromising therapeutic efficacy and with potentially less side effects. There have been 12 published studies comparing once-daily to conventional multiple daily dosing regimens. In all of these studies, once-daily dosing was as effective and no more toxic than multiple daily dosing of the drug. In animal models, rats receiving a single daily dose of aminoglycosides demonstrated less nephrotoxicity and less renal accumulation of the drug than those rats receiving the same total daily dose by a multiple daily dosing schedule. All aminoglycosides may cause or increase neuromuscular blockade.

Dosage Guidelines for Adults and Children

Gentamicin or Tobramycin: 4-6 mg/kg q24h

Amikacin: 15-20 mg/kg q24h

(infused over 30 min.; dilute in 50-100ml D5W or NS)

Dose is based upon ideal body weight (IBW) in kg:

IBW Males: 50+2.3 x (#inches over 5 feet)

IBW Females: 45.5 + 2.3 x (#inches over 5 feet)

Obesity: use IBW + 0.4(Actual BW-IBW)

Creatinine Clearance (ml/min)	Dosing Interval
≥ 60	q24h
40-59	q36h
20-39	q48h
< 20	Avoid once-daily dosing

$$\text{Estimated CrCl (ml/min)} = \frac{(140\text{-age}) \times \text{Weight (Kg)}}{\text{Scr } (\mu\text{mol/L})} \times 1.2 \ (\times 0.85 \text{ if female})$$

Monitoring

It is not necessary to draw standard peak and trough levels. There is no clinical evidence to suggest that adjusting the dosage to achieve a particular target concentration following, or prior to, the drug administration influences outcome in any way with once-daily administration. Monitoring may be required if there is significant changes in renal function.

1) Guidelines for Antimicrobial Use. The Toronto Hospital. 1995: 69-72.

2) Levison, ME, New dosing regimens for aminoglycoside antibiotics. Ann Intern Med 1992; 117: 693-4.

3) Gilbert, DN, Once-daily aminoglycoside therapy. Antimicrob Agents Chemother 1991; 35: 399-405.

4) Sanford, JP, Gilbert DN., Sande, MA. Sanford Guide to Antimicrobial Therapy 1996.

5) Knudson, K. Once daily dosing of aminoglycosides. The Consultant Pharmacist 1995; 10(8): 801-810.

Bibliography

1) American Heart Association recommendations. JAMA 1990; 264:2919-2922.
2) Antibiotic Guidelines Sub-Committee. Antibiotic guidelines. 8th edition. Victorian Medical Postgraduate Foundation Inc.: North Melbourne, Australia. 1994.
3) Arola M, et al. J Pediatr 1990; 116: 697.
4) Balter M, et al. Recommendations on the Management of Chronic Bronchitis. Can Med Assoc J 1994; 151 (suppl): 3-23.
5) Bennett DR, ed. Drug evaluations annual 1996. American Medical Association: Chicago. 1996.
6) Beutner KR, Friedman DJ, Forszpaniak C, et al. Valaciclovir compared with acyclovir for improved therapy for herpes zoster in immunocompetent adults. Antimicrobial Agents Chemotherapy 1995; 39:1546-1553.
7) Boldy D, Skidmore S, Ayres J. Acute bronchitis in the community: clinical features, infective factors, changes in pulmonary function and bronchial reactivity to histamine. Respiratory Medicine 1990; 84:377-385.
8) Breese BB, Denny FW, Dillon, HC, et al. Consensus difficult management problems in children with streptococcal pharyngitis. Pediatr Infect Dis 1985; 4: 10-13.
9) Burrascano JJ. Managing Lyme Disease. 11th edition. The Lyme Disease Network of NJ, Inc.: East Brunswick. 1996.
10) Burtin, et al. Safety of Metronidazole in pregnancy: A Meta-analysis. AM J Obstet Gynecol 1995; 172:525-529.
11) Canada Communicable Disease Report. Statement on management of persons exposed to pertussis and pertussis outbreak control. 1994; 20:193-199.
12) Canada Communicable Disease Report. Pertussis Consensus Conference. 1993; 19-16:124 -36.
13) Canadian Guidelines for the Prevention, Diagnosis, Management and Treatment of Sexually Transmitted Diseases in neonates, children, adolescents and adults. MacDonald N, Bowie W, ed. Laboratory Centre for disease control, Health Protection Branch, Health and Welfare: Ottawa. 1995.
14) Canadian Paediatric Society. How to diagnose and treat Lyme disease in children. CMAJ 1992; 147:169-172.
15) Canadian Paediatric Society. Statement: Chickenpox - Prevention and Treatment. Can J of Paediatrics 1994; 1:88-93.
16) Canadian Paediatric Society. Statement: Tetracycline use in children. 1994 (ID 94-02).
17) 1995 Canadian recommendations for the prevention and treatment of malaria among international travellers. C.A.T.M.A.T. (Committee to Advise on Tropical Medicine and Travel): Ottawa.
18) Centor RM, Witherspoon JM, Dalton HP, et al. The diagnosis of strep throat in adults in the emergency room. Med Dec Making 1981; 1:239-246.
19) Chapman RS, Henderson FW, Clyde WA Jr, et al. The epidemiology of tracheobronchitis in pediatric practice. Amer J Epidemiology 1981; 114:786-797.
20) Clayton MI, Osborne JE, Rutherford D, Rivron RP. A double-blind, randomized, prospective trail of a topical antiseptic versus a topical antibiotic in treatment of otorrhea. Clin Otolaryngol 1990; 15:7-10.
21) Conference de Consensus: Les infections des voies respiratoires. Rev Mal Resp 1992; 9:477-480.
22) Consensus Conference on Lyme Disease. Can J Infect Dis 1991; 2:49-54.

23) Conte JE, Barriere SL. Manual of antibiotics and infectious diseases. 7th edition. Lea & Febiger: Philadelphia. 1992.

24) Coyle PK. Neurologic complications of lyme disease care. Neurologic Aspects of Rheumatic Diseases 1993; 19:993-1002.

25) Del Beccaro MA, et al. J Pediatrics 1992; 120:81.

26) Duerden BI. Guidelines for antimicrobial treatment. South Glamorgan Microbiology Services: U.K. 1993.

27) Durack DR. Prevention of infective endocarditis. NEJM 1995; 332:38-44.

28) Fairbanks D. Pocket guide to antimicrobial therapy in otolaryngology - head and neck surgery. 6th edition. The American Academy of Otolaryngology - Head and Neck Surgery Foundation, Inc.: Virginia. 1993.

29) Farrand RJ. Antimicrobial prescribing guidelines. Bolton Health Authority: U.K. 1993.

30) Forward K, Gold R, Gribble M, et al. Consensus recommendations for management of acute exacerbations of chronic bronchitis. The Can J of Diagnosis 1990; 7:129-139.

31) Humbert, G. French consensus on antibiotherapy of urinary tract infections. Infection 1992; 20 (Suppl. 3):S171-S172.

32) Keystone JS. Malaria update presentation. 1996.

33) Krogh CM ed. Compendium of Pharmaceuticals and Specialties. 31st edition. Canadian Pharmaceutical Association: Ottawa. 1996.

34) Mandell LA, Niederman M. The Canadian Community Acquired Pneumonia Consensus Conference Group. Antimicrobial treatment of community acquired pneumonia in adults: A conference report. Can J Infect Dis 1993; 4:25-8.

35) Marrie TJ. Tuberculosis. In: Gray J, ed. Therapeutic Choices. 1st Edition. CPhA. 1995: 662-668.

36) McKendrick MW, McGill JI, Wood MJ. Lack of effect of acyclovir on post herpetic neuralgia. BMJ 1989; 298:431.

37) The Medical Letter: Handbook of antimicrobial therapy. New Rochelle. 1994.

38) Meyers BR. Antimicrobial therapy guide. 11th edition. Antimicrobial Prescribing, Inc.: Pennsylvania. 1996.

39) Ministry of Ontario. STD treatment guidelines. Government of Ontario: Canada. June, 1992.

40) Murray AE. Antibiotic prescribing guidelines for common infections in general practice and some indications for prophylaxis. Scunthorpe Health Authority: U.K. 1993.

41) Nelson JD. Pocketbook of pediatric antimicrobial therapy. 12th edition. Williams & Wilkins: Baltimore. 1996/97.

42) Orr PH, Scherer K, Macdonald A, Moffatt MEK. Randomized placebo-controlled trials of antibiotics for acute bronchitis: A critical review of the literature. The Journal of Family Practice 1993; 36:507-512.

43) Pennie RA. Mantoux tests. Performing, interpreting, and acting upon them. Can Fam Physician 1995; 41:1025-1029.

44) Piper et al. Prenatal use of metronidazole and birth defects: no association Obstet Gynecol 1993; 82:348-352.

45) Reese RE. A practical approach to infectious diseases. 4th edition. Little, Brown & Company: Toronto. 1996.

46) Rosenfeld RM, Vertrees JE, Carr J, et al. Clinical efficacy of antimicrobial drugs for acute otitis media: Meta-analysis of 5400 children from thirty-three randomized trials. J Pediatr 1994; 124:355-67.

47) Royal College of Dental Surgeons. Recommended antibiotic prophylaxis for dental, oral or upper respiratory tract procedures. 1995.

48) Sanford JP. Guide to antimicrobial therapy. Antimicrobial Therapy Inc.: Dallas. 1996.

49) Saskatchewan Health. Selection of antimicrobial drugs - Saskatchewan Health Formulary. 39th edition. Government of Saskatchewan: Canada. July, 1994.

50) Smith JL, ed. The 1996 formulary of Drugs for Sick Children. 15th Edition. The Hospital for Sick Children: Toronto. 1996.

51) Spotswood L, Spruance MD, Stephen K, et al. A large-scale, placebo-controlled dose-ranging trial of peroral valaciclovir for episodic treatment of recurrent herpes genitalis. Arch Intern Med 1996; 156:1729-1735.

52) Stamm WE, Hooton TM. Management of urinary tract infections in adults. N Engl J Med 1993; 329:1328-34.

53) Swann RA. General practitioner antimicrobial prescribing guidelines. Leicestershire Family Health Services Authority: U.K. 1993.

54) Tyring S, et al. Famciclovir for the treatment of acute herpes zoster: Effects on acute disease and postherpetic neuralgia. Annals of Internal Medicine 1995;123: 89-96.

55) Verheij TJM, Hermans J, Mulder JD. Effects of doxycycline in patients with acute cough and purulent sputum: a double blind placebo controlled trial. British Journal of General Practice 1994; 44:400-404.

56) Wald ER. Sinusitis in children. N Eng J Med 1992; 326:319-323.

57) Wald ER, Chiponis D, Ledesma-Medina J. Comparative effectiveness of amoxicillin and amoxicillin-clavulanate potassium in acute paranasal sinus infections in children: a double-blind, placebo-controlled trail. Pediatrics 1986; 77:795-800.

58) Williams J, Simel D. Does this patient have sinusitis? Diagnosing acute sinusitis by history and physical examination. JAMA 1993; 270:1242-1246.

59) Williams J, Holleman D, Samsa G, Simel D. Randomized controlled trail of 3 vs 10 days of trimethoprim/sulfamethoxazole for acute maxillary sinusitis. JAMA 1995; 273:1015-1021.

60) Wright JR. Traveller's Diarrhea. In: Gray J, ed. Therapeutic Choices. 1st Edition. CPhA. 1995: 662-668.

Index

P

Pelvic inflammatory disease, 59
Peri-anal abscesses, 31
Pertussis, 26
Pharyngitis, 2
Pneumonia, 18, 19, 20, 21, 22, 23, 24, 25, 92
Prostatitis
   Acute, 55
   Chronic, 56
Pyelonephritis, 54

R

Reportable diseases, 84
Rhinitis, 4

S

Shingles, 43
Sinusitis, 12, 13
Strep. throat, 2
Swimmer's ear, 5

T

Toxic shock-like syndrome, 35
Traveller's diarrhea, 73
Tuberculosis, 80

U

Urethritis, 60, 61
Urinary tract infection
   Acute cystitis, 48
   Asymptomatic, 53
   Children, 51
   Chronic, 53
   Complicated, 52

V

Vaginitis, 62
Varicella zoster, 43, 44

W

Whooping cough, 26

COMMENT SHEET

We welcome your participation in the revision to the guidelines by receiving your comments and recommendations on how to improve them.

Item	Yes	No	How Can This Document Be Improved?
1. Concise, easy to understand			
2. Covers most common conditions and circumstances (adult, children etc.)			
3. Relevant to community practice			
4. Relevant to other types of practice.			
5. Are you using the guidelines in your practice?			
6. Are there other guidelines that have more user friendly formats? If so, please list.			

cont...

c
u
t

h
e
r
e

COMMENT SHEET cont...

Item	Yes	No	How Can This Document Be Improved?
7. Useful to have guidelines formatted on computer disk?			
8. Other comments and feedback on any of the specific guidelines.			
9. Recommendations for other guideline topics.			
10. Please note your area of practice (i.e., family medicine, infectious diseases, pediatrics, community pharmacy, etc.)			

Please return to:

Ontario Anti-infective Review Panel, P.O. Box # 60059, 1052 Pape Ave., Toronto, Ontario M4K 3Z3 or Fax (416) 597-8574.

Please provide a return address, fax and telephone number if you would like:
□ **response to your comments**   □ **updates**   □ **guidelines on computer disk**
□ **to participate in a future panel on prescribing guidelines**

THANK YOU
Name: _____
Address: _____
_____
_____
Telephone: _____
Fax: _____